Elastography of the Musculoskeletal System

Salvatore Marsico · Albert Solano
Editors

Elastography of the Musculoskeletal System

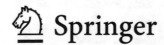 Springer

Editors
Salvatore Marsico
Department of Radiology
Hospital Del Mar
Barcelona, Spain

Albert Solano
Department of Radiology
Hospital Del Mar
Barcelona, Spain

ISBN 978-3-031-31056-0   ISBN 978-3-031-31054-6   (eBook)
https://doi.org/10.1007/978-3-031-31054-6

This Springer imprint is published by the registered company Springer Nature Switzerland AG
The registered company address is: Gewerbestrasse 11, 6330 Cham, Switzerland

Preface

When we accepted Springer's invitation to write this book, we decided that it had to meet several essential requirements. One of them was the choice of world references and, given the authors who have graciously accepted our invitation, we do not doubt that we have succeeded. The choice of chapters has not been random, they have been selected to be of interest in different medical specialties including Rheumatology, Dermatology, Sports Medicine and Rehabilitation, Traumatology, Oncology and Radiology. Considering the diversity of the possible readers, the chapters have been elaborated in a didactic but rigorous way, showing the author's personal experience in the subject. Our greatest achievement would be to get elastography to be considered as another tool in a routine ultrasound study.

We are aware that we have not dealt with all the topics in which elastography can have a wide development and implication in the medical practice, but who knows, maybe there will be the second part of this extraordinary training experience in which we have had the honour to participate.

We have organized a complete review which has as its objective first the exposure of the state of the art regarding this technique in the literature, trying to make what is already known on the subject complete and understandable, and at the same time trying to have a book with clinically practical connotations in the implementation of elastography in the musculoskeletal system and soft tissues.

The book is designed to be useful for both the novice and an experienced ultrasound operator. It is a collection of the experience of our research group and of some of the world's references in elastography with its application in the most advanced ultrasound systems.

First, we have analysed the technical-physical bases of elastography, trying above all to deal with the aspects that are decisive in the diagnostic procedure, the technical appropriateness, with artefacts and technical tricks to have a valid elastographic image.

Secondly, we have tried to treat the pathology of the musculoskeletal system and the soft tissues in a macro-systemic way, with the help of world references on the respective topics.

Each chapter presents a description of the elastographic semiotics of the main pathologies of the musculoskeletal system and soft tissue, images that represent both routine and more complex clinical cases in a practical and schematic way and summary tables on the characteristics in terms of elasticity found in the main pathologies.

Particular attention has been given to the evaluation of the prospects of this imaging method as we know that despite its widespread use, it has areas in which its application is very limited, such as the study of rheumatological and inflammatory articular pathologies and in which our research group, in collaboration with the Rheumatology Department of the Hospital del Mar, believes and tries to develop.

We would like to give our thanks to the patients who have participated and are participating in our research studies, which have allowed this technology to reach routine clinical use.

We want to give a special thanks to the medical and technical, nursing and administrative staff of the Radiology Department of the Hospital del Mar, who have allowed us to easily apply this technique in our clinical routine allowing us to accumulate a remarkable clinical experience in this field, especially in the last 3 years and without which it would have been impossible just to imagine the drafting of this book.

Thanks to the staff of General Electrics for their help in facilitating our studies, especially in the field of technical optimization of the ultrasounds we use and the resolution of artefacts that are critical in our field.

Without the trust that Springer has placed in us, this extraordinary project would not have been possible. We would like to thank the magnificent work done by each of the authors who have participated in the book, and we hope to have the opportunity to collaborate with them again soon.

But above all, we would like to express our most sincere and profound gratitude to our wives, Gaia and Teresa, and to our families for their unconditional and daily encouragement, understanding and infinite tolerance in the face of such a demanding and rewarding experience.

The book is dedicated to them.

Barcelona, Spain   Salvatore Marsico
Barcelona, Spain   Albert Solano

Contents

Abbreviations

2D-THE	2D time-harmonic elastography
ACS	acute compartment syndrome
ACSH	adhesive capsulitis of the shoulder
AOFAS	American Orthopaedic Foot & Ankle Society scores
APL	abductor pollicis longus
ARFI	acoustic radiation force impulse
ATFL	anterior talofibular ligament
BCC	basal cell carcinomas
BoNT-A	botulin toxin A
CAP	controlled attenuation parameter
CHL	coracohumeral ligament
CFL	calcaneofibular ligament
CK	creatine kinase
CMC	carpometacarpal
CP	cerebral palsy
CT	computed tomography
CTS	carpal tunnel syndrome
CUSE	comb-push ultrasound shear elastography
DOMS	delayed onset muscle soreness
DPN	diabetic polyneuropathy
DXA	dual X-ray absorptiometry
EPB	extensor tendons pollicis brevis
ES	elastosonography
ESSDAI	EULAR Sjögren's Syndrome Disease Activity Index scores
ESSPRI	EULAR Sjögren's Syndrome Patient Reported Index
EWGSOP	European Working Group on Sarcopenia in Older People
FNAB	fine-needle aspiration biopsy
FOV	field of view
FPM	flexor pronator muscle
FR	frame rate
HE	harmonic elastography
HIFU	high-intensity focused ultrasound
HMI	harmonic motion imaging
IIM	idiopathic inflammatory myopathies
kPa	kilopascal
LDH	lactate dehydrogenase

LSM	liver stiffness measurement
MAS score	Modified Ashworth Scale
MCL	medial collateral ligament
MCP	metacarpophalangeal
MRI	magnetic resonance imaging
MSGUS	major salivary gland ultrasonography
MTL	multiple tracking location
Non-GA	non-gouty arthritis
NPV	negative predictive value
OA	osteoarthritis
OMERACT US	Outcome Measures in Rheumatoid Arthritis Clinical Trials Ultrasound
PD	power Doppler
PDUS	power Doppler ultrasound
PET	positron emission tomography
PPV	positive predictive value
pSWE	point shear wave elastography
pSS	primary Sjögren's syndrome
PTFL	posterior talofibular ligament
ROI	region of interest
RA	rheumatoid arthritis
RF	radiofrequency
SDUV	shear dispersion ultrasound vibrometry
SE	strain elastography
SFT	solitary fibrous tumours
SLE	systemic lupus erythematosus
SMURG	spatially modulated ultrasound radiation force
SNR	signal-to-noise ratio
SR	strain ratio
SSI	supersonic shear imaging
SSM	spleen stiffness measurement
STL	single tracking location
SWE	shear wave elastosonography
SWW	shear wave velocities
TE	transient elastography
TES	Tsukuba Elasticity Score
WHO	World Health Organization
VA	vibro-acoustography
VISA-A	Victorian Institute of Sport Assessment—Achilles questionnaire
VTQ	virtual touch quantification
UCL	ulnar collateral ligament of the elbow
US	ultrasound

Elastography: Technical Aspects

Salvatore Marsico, José María Maiques, and Albert Solano

1.1 Introduction

The term rheology was coined by Cook Bingham in 1920, inspired by the aphorism of Heraclitus. Rheology is a branch of physics which studies the characteristics of the deformable body including their elasticity, viscosity, plasticity, and fluidity.

An image is a representation of specific properties of a physical object. Medical images are made based on exploiting physical processes as contrast mechanisms. In biomedical ultrasound, the basic contrast mechanism is the acoustic impedance differences between different structures related to the compressibility of tissue [1].

Purely mechanical characterization of materials, based on tensile and compression mechanical testing, has classically been considered the gold standard, although it often involves injury to the material under study. Over the past 30 years, scientists have focused their studies on generating non-invasive techniques to create images based on differences in the stiffness of body tissues.

This imaging modality is known as elasticity imaging or elastography.

The advantages of this modality are that it would be objective, quantitative, examiner-independent, and with high spatial and temporal resolution [2].

Ormachea et al. [3] state that elastography allows a non-invasive way to visualize and quantify the rheology of tissues and internal organs of the body.

A thorough examination and evaluation of changes in the biomechanical qualities of tissues should lead to earlier diagnosis and more effective therapy of diseases, as well as help us to understand the various physiological states of cells, tissues, and organs. For this reason, different authors [4] consider that elastography may represent the most important advance in medical imaging since the invention of Doppler. However, until elastography becomes an additional tool in the ultrasound study of the patient, this statement will not be fully valid (Fig. 1.1).

This chapter will discuss only the physical basis of elastography as applied to ultrasound.

S. Marsico · J. M. Maiques · A. Solano (✉)
Department of Radiology, Hospital del Mar, Passeig
Marítim de la Barceloneta, Barcelona, Spain
e-mail: asolano@psmar.cat

© The Author(s), under exclusive license to Springer Nature Switzerland AG 2023
S. Marsico, A. Solano (eds.), *Elastography of the Musculoskeletal System*,
https://doi.org/10.1007/978-3-031-31054-6_1

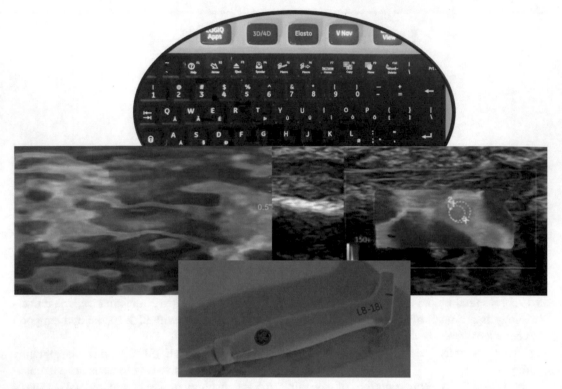

Fig. 1.1 The technique of ultrasound elastography should be valued as an additional tool in any study performed in routine medical practice

1.2 Physics Principles of Ultrasound Elastography

Ultrasound Elastography (USE) is based on the principle that the application of a stress force on a tissue will induce internal displacements intrinsically related to its elastic properties. USE methods vary, but they always involve the same three steps: applying excitation (stress), measuring tissue reaction (strain), and estimating mechanical parameters (Fig. 1.2).

When a material is subjected to stress it will experience strain. Within the elastic limit, strain varies linearly with the applied stress and leads to the definition of the common elastic material properties, which are Young's modulus, bulk modulus, shear modulus, and Poisson's ratio. Additional to these elastic constants there are the longitudinal modulus and transverse modulus that can be determined from the velocity of propagation of longitudinal waves and transverse waves through a solid [5]. The equations that describe physical quantities and laws are called tensor equations. They combine quantities, measured with a number, and represented by scalars, with any special direction [6].

Elastography assesses tissue elasticity, which is the tendency of tissue to resist deformation with an applied force or to resume its original shape after the removal of the force.

In physics, a constitutive equation is a relation between two physical quantities that is specific to a material or substance and approximates the response of that material to external stimuli. The first constitutive equation was developed by Robert Hooke and is known as Hooke's law. It deals with the case of linear elastic materials [7].

$$\text{Hooke's law } \sigma = \lambda \cdot \varepsilon.$$

Stress (σ) is the force per unit area with units of kilopascals. Strain (ε) is the expansion per unit length which is dimensionless.

The elastic modulus (λ) relates stress to strain with units of kilopascals and when compared to

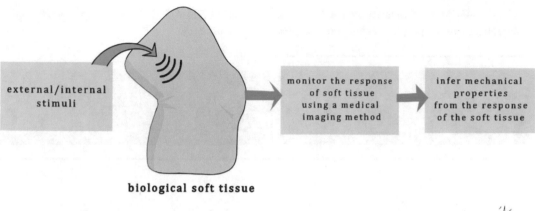

Fig. 1.2 USE always involves the same three steps: applying excitation (stress), measuring tissue reaction (strain), and estimating mechanical parameters

other imaging modalities' properties, the elastic modulus has a greater range, enabling better differentiation between diverse tissues and between normal and pathologic tissues.

There are three types of elastic moduli defined by the method of deformation:

1. *Young's modulus E* is defined by the following equation when a stress (σ) produces a strain (ε), and the strain is perpendicular to the surface.

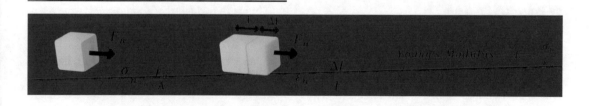

2. *Shear modulus G* is defined by the following equation when shear stress (σ_s) produces a shear strain (ε_s), where shear is tangential to the surface.

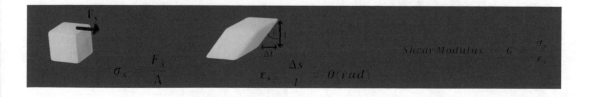

3. *Bulk modulus K* is defined by the following equation when a normal inward force or pressure (σ_B) produces a bulk strain or change in volume (ε_B).

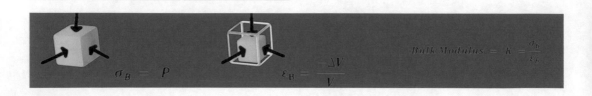

The elastic modulus λ also characterizes the propagation speed of waves:

$$\lambda = c^2 . \rho,$$

where ρ is the material density and c, is the wave speed

Soft tissue material *density* is normally calculated using values from the literature for the type of tissue being studied or is roughly considered to be like water's density (1 g/cm³).

As a solid try to maintain its original volume, the three different forms of deformations and elastic moduli are not independent but have relationships; this endeavour's success is indicated by Poisson's ratio (ν).

There is a direct relationship between the shear and the Young's moduli; $E = 2G (1 + \nu)$, where ν is the Poisson ratio.

Poisson's ratio is a measure of the Poisson effect, the phenomenon in which a material tends to expand in directions perpendicular to the direction of compression. Conversely, if the material is stretched rather than compressed, it usually tends to contract in the direction transverse to the direction of stretching. The Poisson's ratio of a stable, isotropic, linear elastic material must be between −1.0 and +0.5.

Most materials have Poisson's ratio values ranging between 0.0 and 0.5. A perfectly incompressible isotropic material deformed elastically at small strains would have a Poisson's ratio of exactly 0.5 [8] (Fig. 1.3).

Finally, the ratio of axial stress to axial strain in a state of uniaxial deformation is the wave modulus P, also known as the longitudinal modulus or constrained modulus, in linear elasticity.

There are *two types of mechanical wave propagation in ultrasound*: pressure (longitudinal) waves and shear (transverse) waves which propagate independently in the bulk material, interacting only at boundaries (Fig. 1.4).

Longitudinal waves. Longitudinal waves are waves in which the vibration of the medium is parallel to the direction the wave travels and the

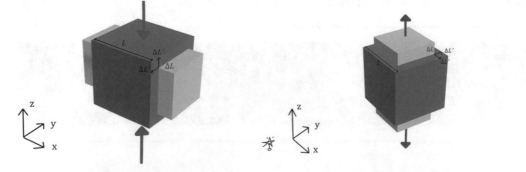

Fig. 1.3 A cube with sides of length L of an isotropic linearly elastic material subject to tension along the *x*-axis, with a Poisson's ratio of 0.5. The blue cube is unstrained, the orange is expanded in the *x* direction by ΔL due to tension, and contracted in the *y* and *z* directions by Δ'L

Fig. 1.4 Types of mechanical wave propagation in ultrasound: pressure (longitudinal) waves and shear (transverse) waves

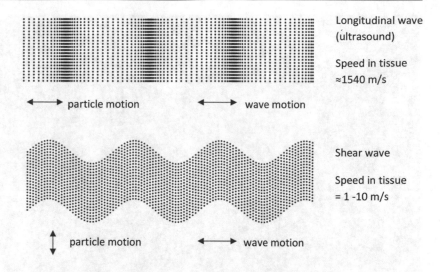

displacement of the medium is in the same (or opposite) direction of the wave propagation. Mechanical longitudinal waves are also called compressional or compression waves because they produce compression and rarefaction when travelling through a medium, and pressure waves, because they produce increases and decreases in pressure. The oscillations in pressure are sinusoidal in nature and are characterized by their frequency, amplitude, and wavelength [9].

They are defined using the bulk modulus where the longitudinal wave speed (c_L) is approximately 1450–1550 m/s.

Whilst longitudinal waves are used in B-mode US, the relatively small differences in wave speed and hence K between different soft tissues do not allow adequate tissue contrast for elastography measurements.

Shear waves have particle motion perpendicular to the direction of wave propagation and are defined using the shear modulus where the shear wave speed (c_S) is approximately 1–10 m/s in soft tissues. Shear wave propagation velocity depends on tissue stiffness. It is well known that biological tissues exhibit a larger attenuation of the shear waves. The amplitude of the shear wave decreases during propagation approximately 10,000 times faster than longitudinal conventional ultrasound waves and Shear waves go through soft tissues at a speed of around a thousand times slower [10].

Shear waves cannot propagate in liquids with zero or very low viscosity; however, they may propagate in liquids with high viscosity This concept is crucial for understanding inflammatory joint pathology, as it will help us to potentially distinguish between synovitis and joint effusion (Fig. 1.5).

The shear moduli of human tissue can span six orders of magnitude, from a few hundred Pa for brain tissue to several GPa for bone and cartilage [11]. Also, the shear moduli of diseased tissues can increase 2–10 fold when compared to healthy baseline values High elasticity contrast for disease states is beneficial in clinical diagnosis but can pose challenges when estimating properties [12]. The low wave speed in soft tissues allows for high differences in shear elastic modulus between tissues, giving suitable tissue contrast for elastography measurements (Fig. 1.6).

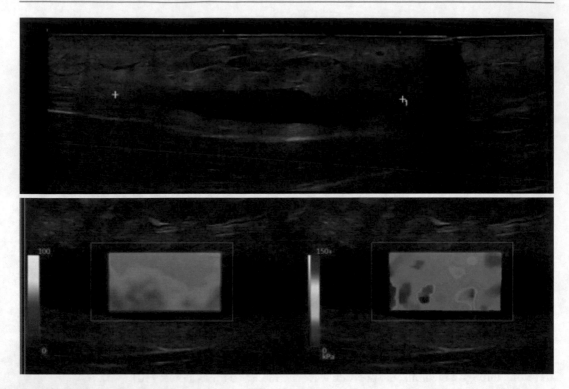

Fig. 1.5 Conventional ultrasound (up) and Shear Wave Elastography (down) images showing the transmissibility of Shear Waves in viscous liquids (infected seroma)

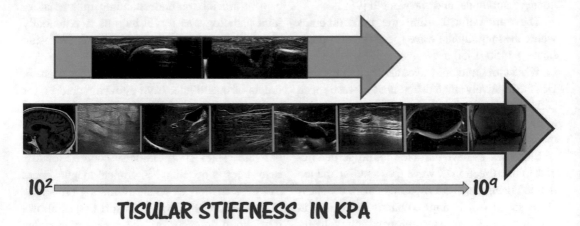

Fig. 1.6 In the evaluation of the mechanical properties of the different human tissues the shear elastic moduli play an important role for two reasons; firstly because of the enormous difference in its value between the different tissues and secondly because of the variation that can occur within the same tissue when it is affected by pathology or when it is within the normal range

1.3 Ultrasound Elastography Technique

The key steps involved in an elastography method are:

1. A target soft tissue is subjected to external or internal stimulation.
2. Monitoring is done of the soft tissue's reactions, including its static and/or dynamic deformation behaviours.
3. Using inverse analysis, it is, therefore possible to deduce from the measured responses the mechanical characteristics of the soft tissue.

To make the processing and interpretation of data and images more straightforward, commercially available USE modes rely on several presumptions about the tissue material being studied [13]. Core assumptions are that the tissue is:

- Linear: resulting strain linearly increases as a function of incremental stress,
- Elastic: tissue deformation is not dependent on stress rate, and tissue returns to its original non-deformed equilibrium state.
- Isotropic: the tissue is symmetrical/homogeneous and responds to stress the same from all directions.
- Incompressible: the overall volume of tissue remains the same under stress applied.

But the real situation is that the biomechanics of tissue can exhibit anisotropic, viscous, and nonlinear behaviour, and these properties will differ depending on the direction, extent, and rate of deformation [3].

The majority of elastography efforts have concentrated on recovering the linear properties of tissues, ignoring their nonlinear behaviour, which is seen in some neoplasms and is characterized by malignant tissue's tendency to harden more with increasing strain.

The development, assessment, and advancement of elastography methods depend critically on continuum mechanics, which also makes it possible to predict how biological soft tissue will react to a static load or a dynamic stimulus. The field of classical mechanics known as continuum mechanics [14, 15] examines the mechanical behaviour of materials that are modelled as continuous masses as opposed to discrete particles. Since the continuum model postulates that the substance of an object completely fills the area it occupies, we define an object as continuous if it can be continuously divided into tiny pieces with attributes identical to those of the original material. A basic principle of contemporary physics, atomic structure, and interactions between atoms are not considered in continuum mechanics. Continuum mechanics is based on a series of axioms or basic principles whose exhaustive review is not feasible in this chapter, however, I would like to mention in a very brief way the material frame indifference principle (MFI), whose interpretation has varied in the last decades due to its vague mathematical definition.

Mathematically, the material frame indifference principle can be stated as the invariance of the constitutive function under frame change. Liu or Sampaio [16], however, claim that the ultimate meaning of the IFM is the simple idea that material properties are independent of observers.

An inverse problem in science is the process of calculating from a set of observations the causal factors that produced them and many important inverse problems in engineering and science are ill-posed.

French mathematician Jacques Hadamard defined the concept of a "well-posed problem" in the twentieth century. He thought that mathematical representations of physical phenomena should include:

1. A solution exists and is unique.
2. The solution's behaviour changes continuously with the initial conditions.

An inverse problem is ill-posed if one of the Hadamard properties is not respected.

Besides linear elastic parameters, it has been demonstrated that hyperelastic, viscoelastic, and anisotropic elastic parameters of soft tissues may be inferred using different inverse methods reported in recent years [17].

1.4 Primary Categories of Ultrasonic Elastography Techniques

Elastography is generally classified by the imaging modality, the measured physical quantity, and the applied stimulus or load that is utilized. As mentioned in the introduction, we will focus exclusively on ultrasound techniques. The way to categorize the more widely used approaches is by the class of applied stimulus: quasi-static and dynamic. Continual (harmonic) or transient stimuli are the two main categories within dynamic approaches [3, 17] (Figs. 1.7 and 1.8).

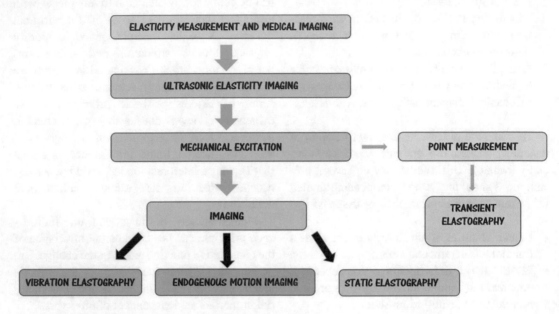

Fig. 1.7 Ultrasound elasticity imaging by a mechanical excitation

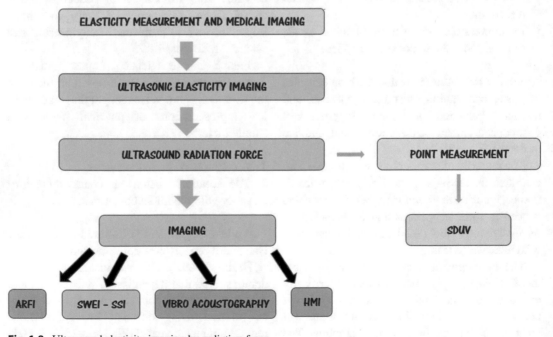

Fig. 1.8 Ultrasound elasticity imaging by radiation force

We would like to briefly discuss vibration amplitude sonoelastography (VASE), which is regarded as the original elasticity imaging technique and the first dynamic elasticity imaging. Lerner et al. [18] introduced this method for the detection of hard lesions in relatively soft tissue. Vibration amplitude sonoelastography entails the application of a continuous low-frequency vibration (40–1000 Hz) to excite internal shear waves within the tissue of interest The main idea is to send low-amplitude and low-frequency shear waves through deep organs (with displacements below 0.1 mm and then use advanced colour Doppler imaging techniques to display the vibration response in real time. Vibration above a predetermined threshold (in the 2-μm range) resulted in a saturated colour in these images.

The eigenmode pattern would be locally perturbed by lesions, and from the patterns at discrete eigenfrequencies, the background Young's modulus could be determined. Therefore, vibration elastography could be used to perform tasks for both quantitative and relative image contrast detection [19].

1.4.1 Quasi-Static Ultrasound Elastography Techniques

There are two approaches for strain imaging using ultrasound:

1.4.1.1 Strain Elastography (SE)

Two-dimensional (2D) tissue strain estimates were introduced by Ophir et al. (1991) and are considered a qualitative or semi-quantitative technique based on the application of compressive waves on tissues [3]. In strain elastography, by means of manual compression with the transducer itself or by means of a specially designed mechanism or by taking advantage of the changes inherent in cardiac movement, respiration, or the beating of blood vessels, a small tissue movement is generated, which most authors estimate to be approximately 2%.

Subsequently, by cross correlating the pre- and post-deformed RF echo frames we determine the displacement generated in the tissue in the axial axis (Fig. 1.9).

Given a certain amount of applied stress, softer tissues have more deformation and, therefore, experience larger strain than stiffer tissues (Fig. 1.10).

The strain *measurements are displayed as a semitransparent colour map called an elastogram, which is overlaid on the B-mode image. Although there is a strong* tendency towards uniformity of scale, it should be noted that the scale of the elastogram may change depending on the firm. Low strain (stiff tissue) is typically shown in red, whereas high strain (soft tissue) is typically shown in blue (Fig. 1.11).

Although there have been numerous studies for the application of semi-quantitative assessment (like the Tsukuba score) of tissue stiffness using

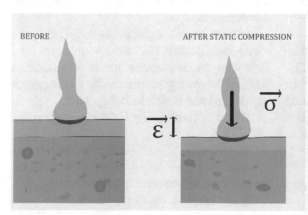
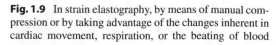
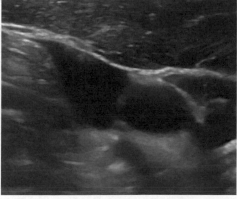

Fig. 1.9 In strain elastography, by means of manual compression or by taking advantage of the changes inherent in cardiac movement, respiration, or the beating of blood vessels, a small tissue movement is generated that can be measured in axial plane

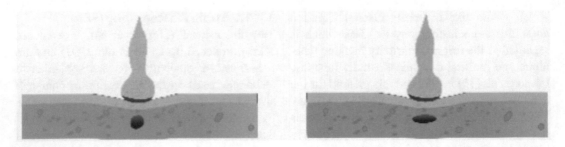

Fig. 1.10 Given a certain amount of applied stress, softer tissues have more deformation and, therefore, experience larger strain than stiffer tissues

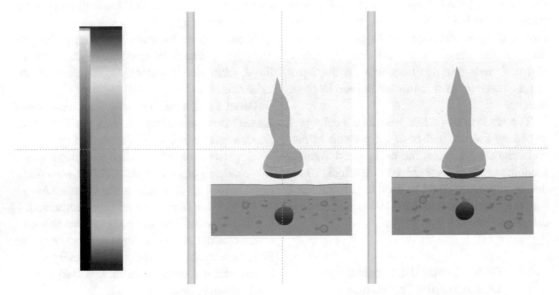

Fig. 1.11 Low strain (stiff tissue) is typically shown in red, whereas high strain (soft tissue) is typically shown in blue in the elastogram colour map

strain elastography, there exists no, linear relationship between degree of tissue stiffness and brightness/colour code on the strain elastogram [20].

The strain ratio a pseudo-quantitative measurement is the ratio of strain measured in adjacent (usually normal) reference tissue region of interest (ROI) to strain measured in a target lesion [4]. A strain ratio > 1 indicates that the target lesion compresses less than the normal reference tissue, indicating lower strain and greater stiffness (Fig. 1.12).

Recently an acoustic coupler with a known Young's modulus [21] has been developed for a more consistent strain ratio measurement reference and was shown to be reproducible

and to correlate with qualitative elastography measurements.

Another technical factor to consider is the elastogram quality indicator, which can vary depending on the manufacturer but always show whether the elastogram obtained is valid or not as highlighted and explained in Fig. 1.13.

The main disadvantages of this technique are:

1. The validity of the elastogram is compromised when evaluating structures with significant bone projections since it is challenging to apply uniform compression (Maltese cross artefact) [22].
2. Even with a homogeneous stiff tissue, the stress conveyed to the tissue will decrease

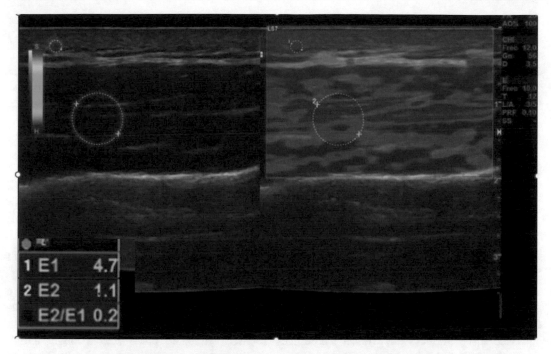

Fig. 1.12 The strain ratio is the ratio of strain measured in adjacent reference tissue region of interest (ROI) to strain measured in a target lesion. A strain ratio > 1 indicates that the target lesion compresses less than the normal reference tissue, indicating lower strain and greater stiffness

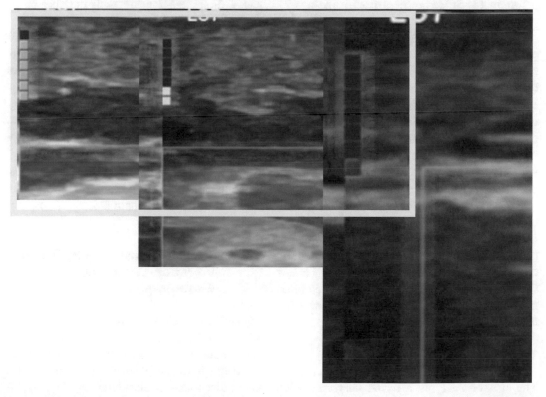

Fig. 1.13 Elastogram quality indicator: The colour of these indicators, which are on the left side, ranges from red to green. The elastogram is invalid if the indicator is red. On the other side, the measurement will be more accurate the greener the indicator is

with increasing distance, resulting in a lesser deformation in the area furthest from the transducer [17].

3. Measurements in both modes are very subjective due to the intrinsic variability of physiologic motion when utilized as a stimulus and the difficulty in controlling the amplitude of the applied stress using operator-dependent manual compression.

4. The degree of stress created by an operator can cause strain concentration artefacts to form around certain structures, which subsequently distort the strain field and produce artefacts in images or inaccurate measurements.

5. Another artefact, called the egg-shell effect is seen as a falsely high tissue stiffness in a necrotic area within a hard lesion [22].

6. Nonlinearity of the mechanical property of tissue also produces an artefact, more the stress applied, the greater the stiffness of tissue, represented as an exponential relationship in mathematical terms. This type of artefact is called prestress artefact [22].

Tension elastography is a variation of compression elastography, with tissue strain measured in response to an internally generated tensile stress, which has been validated recently ex vivo Tensile force is created by voluntary isometric muscle contraction, whereas the generated force is measured externally using a dynamometer and data acquisition system. When compared with compression sonoelastography, tension elastography provides quantitative information related to tissue elasticity (elastic modulus), which is relevant as the primary function of tendons is to transmit tensile force from muscle to bone. Although this technique is not yet commercially available, it holds great promise as a new functional imaging test, which may guide treatment for tendinopathies and other chronic tendon disorders [10].

1.4.1.2 Acoustic Radiation Force Impulse (ARFI) Strain Imaging

The use of ARF as a tissue characterization modality was proposed by Sugimoto et al. (1990) as a laboratory system and the use of ARFI in an imaging system with estimates of displacements from deep internal tissue was described by Nightingale (1999) [3, 13, 23].

The mechanical excitation used to cause tissue motion in ARFI is given with temporal and spatial precision using impulsive, focused acoustic radiation force (ARF), setting it apart from competing strain elastography imaging techniques. An advantage of ARFI imaging versus compression elastography is that the force is applied directly to the targeted tissue, eliminating problems with indirect force coupling and decreasing the stresses required to generate appropriate contrast of mechanical features.

One ultrasound transducer is used for both producing impulsive ARF and detecting the generated displacements in ARFI imaging. The impulsive ARF excitation force, which is a crucial part of ARFI imaging, is supplied by a focused ultrasonic pulse with a longer length and/or higher acoustic power than typical B-mode imaging pulses. The tissue displacement response has an inverse relationship with tissue stiffness and a direct relationship with the size of the applied force [24, 25].

Acoustic radiation force impulse (ARFI) strain imaging achieves finer spatial resolution and is therefore relevant for applications in which structural information is important.

1.5 Shear Wave Imaging

Currently, the largest group of techniques in elastography employ shear wave phenomena associated with transient and harmonic approaches.

1.5.1 Transient Elastography (TE) or Vibration-Controlled Elastography

Matias Fink et al. (1999) and Sandrin et al. (2003) advocated the application of TE as a tissue characterization modality as a laboratory system and imaging system, respectively. It is important to know that transient elastography refers specifically to transient elastic imaging techniques in which transient shear waves are mechanically

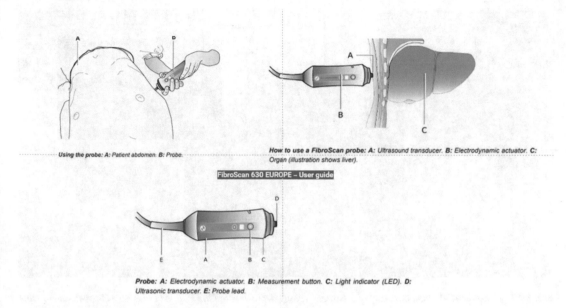

Fig. 1.14 FibroScan® technique and application. Courtesy of Echosens

induced, although transient elastic imaging refers to elastography techniques that are based on the use of transient shear waves [3, 26]. The technological development of this technique is related to Green's function, a powerful mathematical tool. By using transient stimulation, transient elastography minimizes interfering nodes within the medium under study and enables the separation of compression and shear waves [26].

The commercialization of FibroScan® started in December 2003 and currently is the most widely used and validated technique for the assessment of liver fibrosis [27] (Figs. 1.14 and 1.15).

The ultrasound transducer and a vibrator employed during the procedure must be situated on the same axis (reflection mode). The reflection mode ensures a perfect alignment of the ultrasound and shear wave axis of propagation which means that only purely longitudinal displacements can be measured with this setup.

Controlling the shear wave frequency is essential since the viscoelastic parameters of soft tissues are frequency dependent as example the stiffness of a fresh liver can vary between 2 kPa at 50 Hz and 10 kPa at 400 Hz [26].

This technique assesses three parameters:

1. *Liver stiffness measurement* (LSM). Liver stiffness measurement shows excellent results

in the estimation of liver cirrhosis and is a key biomarker for liver diseases and a prognostic factor for cirrhosis.
2. *Controlled attenuation parameter* (CAP). The CAP reflects the degree of fatty infiltration of the organ (steatosis).
3. *Spleen stiffness measurement* (SSM). Finally, the alteration of SSM is related in recent studies to the existence of grade 3 or 4 oesophageal varices.

There have been developments in both one- and two-dimensional TE. The vibration frequency in the one-dimensional TE is as low as 50 Hz, and the tracking ultrasonography has a frame rate of more than 1000 frames per second. In contrast, the two-dimensional TE develops a programmable ultrasound electronic device to accomplish ultrafast imaging, and the raw data are recorded at a frame rate of over 5000 per second [7].

1.5.2 ARF-Based Shear Wave Elastography (SWE)

Radiation force-based elastography techniques exhibit depth- and frequency-dependent bias. The following variables affect the frequency con-

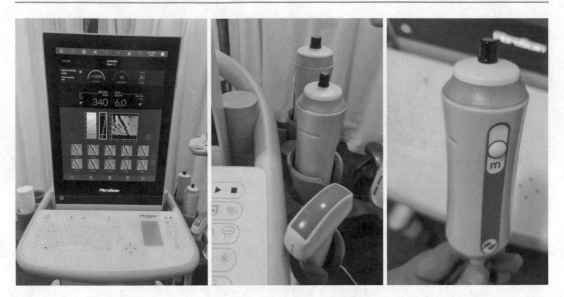

Fig. 1.15 FibroScan®Probes. *Courtesy of gastroenterology department of the Parc de Salut Mar (Barcelona—Spain)*

tent of the shear waves caused by the radiation force [24, 25]:

1. The measurement's depth, as the ultrasound's frequency content varies with depth because of the frequency dependence of the attenuation at the ultrasonic frequencies. In general, in vivo radiation force is mainly related to attenuation in soft tissues (about 0.3–1.0 dB/cm/MHz).
2. The ultrasonic transducer's centre frequency.
3. The length of the ultrasonic transducer's excitation and the radiation force's effect on the tissue's stiffness at the push point.

1.5.3 Point Shear Wave Elastography (pSWE)

Point shear wave also known as quantitative ARF, produces a focused, short-duration ultrasound beam that is directed into a small, localized area (1 cm^3) at a specific depth in the tissue. This technique results in the displacement of the targeted area along the axis of the ultrasound beam that can be detected. The elasticity for the focal area is calculated using the displacement over the time of ARFI stimuli, including the maximum displacement, the time to reach the maximum

displacement, and the relaxation time of the total recovery from the displacement [28].

Most of the published articles focus on comparing this technique with transient elastography in the assessment of liver involvement (fibrosis). The great advantage of pSWE is that it can select the area to be studied and thus avoid structures such as large vessels or dilated bile ducts that affect its measurement and that obesity or the existence of ascites alter less the assessment of hepatic stiffness.

Their main drawback is that the pSWE technique is not a real-time technique as well as the small area to be studied [22].

1.5.4 Shear Wave Elasticity Imaging and ARF Impulse

The shear wave elasticity imaging (SWEI) approach was developed by Sarvazyan et al. in 1998.

On commercial diagnostic ultrasound systems, a method of generating shear waves relies on the phenomenon of acoustic radiation force. This is a body force associated with the propagation of an acoustic wave in an absorptive medium. The direction of the force is in the direction of the flow of acoustic energy. For a weakly focused

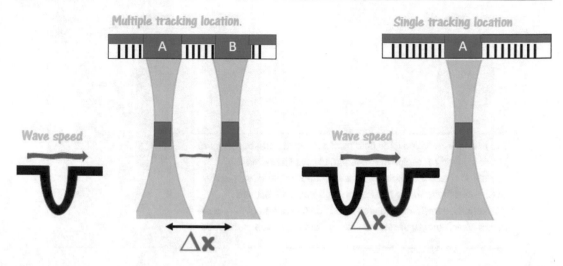

Fig. 1.16 Shear wave elasticity imaging (SWEI)

ultrasound beam of intensity (I), the associated acoustic radiation force F is given by:

$$F = \frac{2\alpha I}{c_L}$$

where α is the absorption coefficient, I the temporal average intensity, and c_L is the specd of sound (Fig. 1.16).

In soft tissues, the variations of cL and α are small compared to the variations in I that can be achieved by focusing. We can thus generate force distributions in tissue in equal proportion to our ability to shape the intensity of an ultrasound beam [25]. High-intensity ultrasound tone bursts with durations of 10^{-5} to 10^{-3} s are thus able to be used to generate localized body forces that act as shear wave sources, a method called acoustic radiation force impulse. (ARFI). Here the term "impulse" is used to imply that the duration of force application is short (a few hundred microseconds long) compared with the timescale of the mechanical response (on the order of milliseconds) of the tissue [25]. The generated waves' amplitudes are small—less than 100 μm —but sufficient for in vivo ultrasonographic measurement [25].

The speed of the shear wave as it propagates away from the source can be measured by timing its arrival at two or more "gates or points" a known distance apart. We will refer to this approach, involving the timing of shear arrival at several locations, as the multiple tracking location (MTL) method. Examples of MTL methods include shear dispersion ultrasound vibrometry, (SDUV), supersonic shear wave imaging (SSI), and ARFI shear wave elastography (ARFI-SWE) (Fig. 1.17) [25].

A complementary approach is to be implemented, which we call a single tracking location (STL).

1.5.5 Supersonic Shear Imaging

Bercoff et al. provided the first description of the supersonic shear imaging (SSI) technique [24]. The uniqueness of this SWEI is characterized by the combination of acoustic radiation force excitation with ultrafast ultrasound imaging of the ensuing shear waves. The following is a brief explanation of the three steps involved in this technique:

1. Excitation by acoustic radiation force. The SSI technique uses radiation force to excite the medium. The radiation pressure is a force that originates from the momentum transfer between a wave and its propagation medium. The acoustic radiation force generates a mechanical force at a distance proportional to the square of the ultrasound amplitude a focusing law is used to locally raise the ampli-

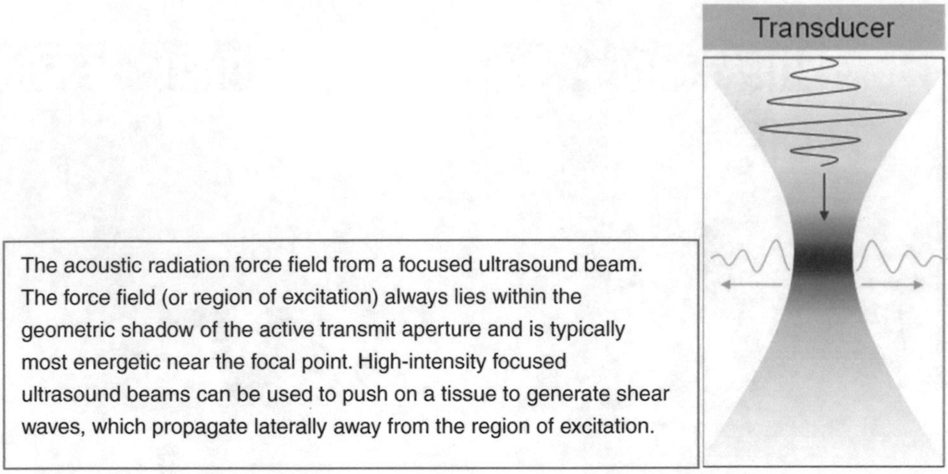

The acoustic radiation force field from a focused ultrasound beam. The force field (or region of excitation) always lies within the geometric shadow of the active transmit aperture and is typically most energetic near the focal point. High-intensity focused ultrasound beams can be used to push on a tissue to generate shear waves, which propagate laterally away from the region of excitation.

Fig. 1.17 Acoustic radiation force impulse

tude of the ultrasonic waves to generate a peak force at a precise point.

The amplitude of this wave is quite low and, in addition, decreases sharply during propagation. The idea behind SSI is to focus the ultrasound on various depths consecutively. As the speed at which the shear wave source is moved in depth is higher than the shear wave rate of the medium, it will create a supersonic regime and a Mach cone. The interference of the shear waves created by each focusing allows one to create a quasi-plane shear wave that greatly reduces the total ultrasound focusing time in the medium and thus reducing the risk of overheating or cavitation.

2. Ultrasound imaging. It has been necessary to develop an imaging mode capable of making several thousand images per second to follow the shear wave in this condition. The SSI technique uses ultrafast imaging by illuminating the medium with an ultrasonic plane wave to obtain an excellent temporal resolution The last step to be able to follow the shear wave is to measure the displacement of the tissue from the ultrafast movie for this purpose, the technique known as ultrasonic speckle interferometry has been developed.

3. Shear Wave Speed Mapping. One possible way to map the shear wave speed in tissues is

to use a time-of-flight algorithm and an intuitive way to find the time that the shear wave travels between two spatial points. Three match cones are needed to properly construct the image and thus be able to infer in a precise way the mechanical properties of the object under study. The Mach cone produced in SWE has the advantage of being less susceptible to decay, allowing better depth penetration (up to 8 cm) [22].

1.5.6 Vibro-acoustography

Vibro-Acoustography (VA) uses the acoustic response of a tissue or object to a vibration created by the ultrasonic radiation force as a non-invasive imaging tool to determine its mechanical properties [29–31]. The VA technique can be summarized in three steps:

1. A localized oscillating force is applied to the tissue to cause vibration.
2. The sound produced by the vibrating tissue is recorded.
3. An image is produced using the recorded acoustic signal.

VA produces a modulated ultrasonic radiation force and an acoustic field by focusing two ultrasound beams at slightly different frequencies on a

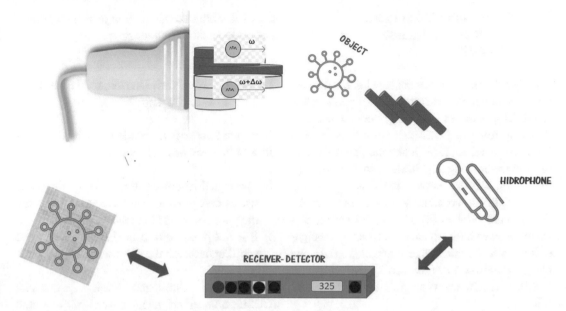

Fig. 1.18 Vibro-acoustography. By concentrating two ultrasound beams at marginally different frequencies on a single region, VA creates an acoustic field and a modulated ultrasonic radiation force. A hydrophone placed nearby collects sound emissions to create an image

single area. Posteriorly, a hydrophone placed nearby obtains acoustic emissions to form an image (Fig. 1.18). The two most important features of the VA image are its high contrast and speckle free. Speckle reduces the contrast of ultrasound images and small structures such as microcalcifications.

The main clinical application of this imaging technology is in young women with high or moderate risk of breast cancer and dense breasts because it has the highest potential for the detection of microcalcifications.

Its major disadvantages are:

1. Lesions that are quite proximal to the chest wall cannot be studied.
2. The length of the study and the patient's pain during picture acquisition.

1.5.7 Harmonic Motion Imaging

Elisa Konofagou et al. devised localized harmonic imaging (HMI) in 2003 [32, 33].

HMI is a radiation force-based elasticity imaging that combines the advantages of diagnostic ultrasound (high spatial and temporal resolution) with the advantages of radiation force-based elasticity imaging (sensitive, reliable, stiffness-based measurements at large depths). HMI utilizes the ultrasound beam to induce oscillatory displacements in the focal area but does not require any direct contact, alignment, or external tissue deformation to infer their mechanical properties.

HMIFU denotes the seamless application of HMI to HIFU (High-Intensity Focused Ultrasound) monitoring. This technique utilizes the same ultrasound beam before, during, and after HIFU treatment. For detecting the changes in tissue elasticity during HIFU treatment, some ultrasound-based elasticity imaging techniques have been developed, including quasi-static elastography, supersonic shear imaging (SSI), acoustic radiation force imaging (ARFI), and HMI.

HMI can differentiate the margins of the treated tumour and thus know in real time the success of the therapy [34].

1.5.8 "Spatially Modulated Ultrasound Radiation Force" (SMURF)

As its acronym states, the concept behind the spatially modulated ultrasound radiation force (SMURF), is to use a spatially variable acoustic radiation force to generate a shear wave with a known wavelength [25]. It was the first method to use single-tracking localization in the development of shear wave elasticity imaging. Wavelength is commonly designated by the Greek letter lambda (λ) The spatial period of a periodic wave or the distance between two neighbouring wave points that correspond to the same phase is referred to as its wavelength in physics. The inverse of the wavelength is called the spatial frequency.

Once it has been generated, this wave's speed can be determined by measuring its frequency f and applying the formula $c = \lambda f$. Assuming linear propagation of the shear wave, its frequency does not change as it propagates. The size of the zone of excitation affects the spatial resolution associated with SMURF [35]. Reducing the extent of the zone of excitation is necessary to improve the spatial resolution of the shear wave speed estimation. The applicability of SMURF is limited to cases where the viscoelasticity of the medium does not inhibit the generation of shear waves of the desired spatial frequency.

1.5.9 Comb-Push Ultrasound Shear Elastography

There are two critical problems with traditional ultrasonic shear wave elastography:

1. The signal-to-noise ratio (SNR) of the shear waves decreases as one advances away from the push beam due to greater attenuation.
2. It is not possible to establish the shear wave speed underneath the shear wave source zone.

Comb-push Ultrasound Shear Elastography (CUSE), a novel technology created by Song et al [36]. in 2003, relies on the employment of several shear wave sources within the tissue. A crucial balance needs to be struck between the two since the shear wave energy of each source is inversely proportional to the total number of sources. Each push beam produces two shear waves propagating in opposite directions away from the push beam. The shear waves from different push beams interfere with each other and eventually fill the entire FOV. The most useful approach for getting rid of interference artefacts is using directional filters [37] (Fig. 1.19).

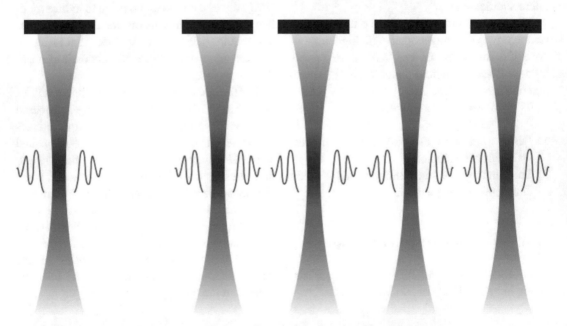

Fig. 1.19 Comparison of single push beams and simultaneous pushing beams in a comb-like pattern

There are three different CUSE modes: focused, unfocused, and marching comb-push, depending on the depth of the area to be explored. The same author has created an even more sophisticated mode called "rain-push" CUSE, which simultaneously distributes numerous shear wave sources at various axial and lateral positions [38].

1.5.10 Harmonic SWE

Another broad category of elastography uses continuous wave external vibration sources and can be classified as harmonic elastography (HE). HE approaches apply a low frequency and a spatially localized sinusoidal mechanical source. The phase and amplitude of the propagating shear waves are estimated by applying similar techniques to those used in colour Doppler imaging [3].

1.5.11 Vibro-Elastography

Vibro-elastography is an extension of static elastography and was developed by Emre Turgay and Rob Rohling. The method consists of applying multi-frequency broadband low-frequency (typically <30 Hz z frequency, 0–3 mm amplitude) compression waves to tissue by an external vibration source. The RF data, collected at the approximate rate of 40 fps, was processed to compute the tissue motion resulting from the applied compression. A measure of strain energy was computed in the frequency domain to show tissue stiffness contrast.

The regional CNR of VE images is significantly higher than that of B-mode. Studies using this technique have been basically oriented towards prostatic [39] and uterine pathology [40], but very few recent articles have been published on it.

1.5.12 Crawling Waves Elastography

The use of crawling waves was first described in 2004 by Wu et al. [41]. It was shown that crawl-ing waves could be used to accurately derive Young's modulus of materials Estimators of shear wave speed and the shear wave attenuation are derived by Hoyt et al. [42].

The term "crawling waves" comes from the useful fact that by implementing a slight frequency difference, on the order of 0.1 Hz, between the two parallel sources, the interference pattern will move across the imaging plane at a speed controlled by the sources [43]. Thus, the crawling waves are readily visualized by conventional Doppler imaging scanners at typical Doppler frame rates; another advantage of crawling waves is that the region of interest excited between the two sources is large. The implementation of scanning probes can be accomplished by utilizing a pair of miniature vibration external sources.

1.5.13 2D Time-Harmonic Elastography (2D-THE)

The method requires single- or multi-frequency external vibrations devices incorporated into the patient bed that generates a shear wave that propagates in multiple directions. These vibrators have been demonstrated to be an efficient way to stimulate tissues in almost all organs and regions of the body. Again, the process consists of three basic steps:

1. For tissue stimulation in the lower-frequency range, a multi-harmonic waveform was designed, which was composed of different frequencies.
2. Raw radiofrequency data were acquired over 1 s at a frame rate (FR) of 80 Hz.
3. The flowchart of the post-processing algorithm is very complicated by referring the interested reader to the original article by Tzschatzsch [44, 45].

The main advantage of this technique is that it allows the evaluation of larger and deeper areas than other SWEI techniques.

1.5.14 Reverberant Shear Wave Elastography

The presence of reflected waves, from organ boundaries and internal inhomogeneities, may cause modal patterns applying continuous waves or backward travelling waves in transient waves. To overcome this problem, reverberant shear wave elastography (SWE) was proposed as an alternative method which applies the concept of a narrow band random isotropic field of shear waves within the tissue.

Like 2D Time Harmonic Elastography external mechanical vibrators (frequency 40–700 Hz) are used and are situated on the same research bed. The reverberant shear wave field can be described as the superposition of plane shear waves propagating in random directions and at least 60 incident plane waves were necessary to generate a reverberant shear wave field. This new method establishes a profusion of shear waves propagating in different directions, incorporating shear wave reflections from boundaries and inhomogeneities.

One advantage of using RSWE is that it produces stronger shear waves at deeper tissue regions of interest (~16 cm depth), and it can provide additional parameters such as the evolution of SWS as a function of frequency (dispersion). In summary, RSWE is an approach that overcomes some major limitations of current elastography: by incorporating reflections and deep penetration of shear waves, avoiding the need for prior knowledge of wave propagation direction, and by minimizing the effects of surface acoustic waves.

I refer the interested reader to the articles provided by Ormachea, Zvietcovich, and Parker [45, 46, 47].

We provide a chronology of the development of elastographic imaging methods over the past 30 years as a summary (Fig. 1.20).

2D SWE generates a colour-coded map in a 2D region of interest and provides the user with a quantitative measurement. It is therefore essential to carry out the study in a rigorous manner and only perform the measurement when strict quality criteria are met in the image obtained (Figs. 1.21 and 1.22).

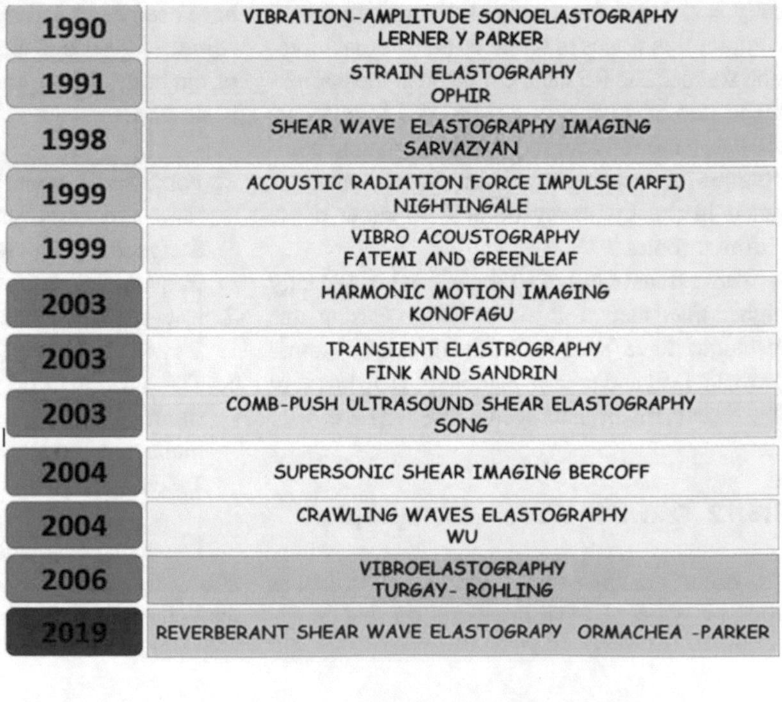

Fig. 1.20 Chronology of the development of elastographic imaging methods over the past 30 years

1990	VIBRATION-AMPLITUDE SONOELASTOGRAPHY LERNER Y PARKER
1991	STRAIN ELASTOGRAPHY OPHIR
1998	SHEAR WAVE ELASTOGRAPHY IMAGING SARVAZYAN
1999	ACOUSTIC RADIATION FORCE IMPULSE (ARFI) NIGHTINGALE
1999	VIBRO ACOUSTOGRAPHY FATEMI AND GREENLEAF
2003	HARMONIC MOTION IMAGING KONOFAGU
2003	TRANSIENT ELASTROGRAPHY FINK AND SANDRIN
2003	COMB-PUSH ULTRASOUND SHEAR ELASTOGRAPHY SONG
2004	SUPERSONIC SHEAR IMAGING BERCOFF
2004	CRAWLING WAVES ELASTOGRAPHY WU
2006	VIBROELASTOGRAPHY TURGAY- ROHLING
2019	REVERBERANT SHEAR WAVE ELASTOGRAPY ORMACHEA -PARKER

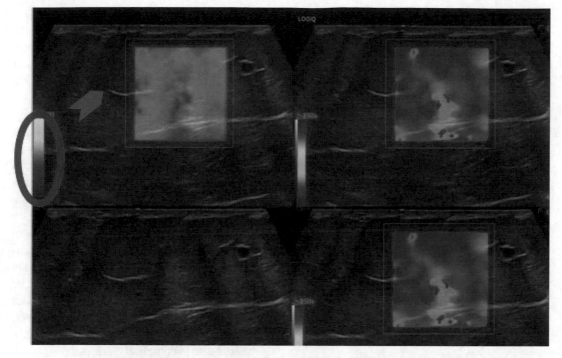

Fig. 1.21 A fundamental characteristic of SWEI is to objectively provide a value of the stiffness of the tissues as an expression of their mechanical properties. However, this value will only be representative if the measurement is performed according to the quality criteria established by the equipment. In this way, in our equipment, the values obtained on red areas in the quality indicator will not be valid or, in other words, the pale yellow or white areas will be the optimal ones in the measurement of the stiffness of tissue

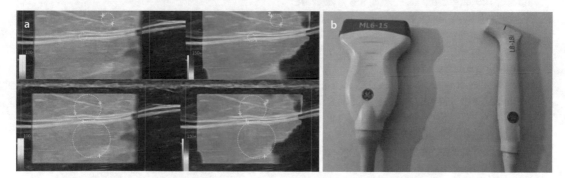

Fig. 1.22 There is controversy about what should be the optimal size of the region of interest on which to measure the stiffness or velocity of the tissue

Therefore, we must ask ourselves the following questions:

1. Is the elastogram obtained valid? All the equipments have an image quality indicator that varies substantially between the different commercial firms. We can only perform the measurement if we are in the quality range set by the manufacturer.

2. The measurement is performed in the right area. With the B-Mode image for guidance, the user can adjust the size and position of the ROI to align with the anatomy of interest.

3. What should be the size of the ROI? It will be determined by the area to be studied (Fig. 1.22a) and the transducer used (Fig. 1.22b). There is no consensus on a specific size. Kot et al. studied the impact of ROI size on quantitative elasticity

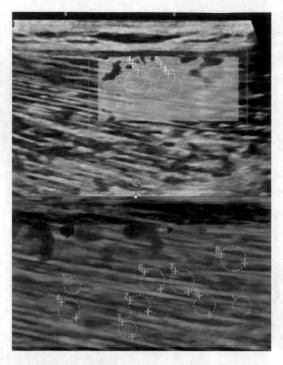

Fig. 1.23 It is accepted that a minimum of three measurements should be made and it is advisable to make five whenever possible

values in a musculotendinous environment [48]. Indeed, the larger the ROI size, the greater the chance of including stiffer structures (fascia, dense collagen fibre). It is recommended to choose a size that reduces the possibility of including artefacts. In the case of heterogeneity of the lesion, it is recommended to measure the different areas with an adjusted ROI [49, 50].

This will depend on the structure to be studied and the transducer used.

Generally, it should be sufficiently adjusted to not include structures that alter the average value of the same and in the case of very heterogeneous structures, measurements should be made on each of the differentiated zones.

What number of measurements should be performed? Again, there is no broad consensus on this issue except for liver assessment.

(a) The guidelines have recommended obtaining a minimum of three acquisitions and using the mean value of the acquisitions as representative of stiffness. We suggest obtaining up to five acquisitions to better judge the variability between measurements (Fig. 1.23).

4. It is recommended to use the IQR/M as a quality factor: it should be ≤30% when the median value is given in kPa and ≤15% when the median value is given in m/s. This cut-off value may vary depending on the anatomical area explored. The recommendation is to try to keep it as low as possible.

5. Measurements should be performed on one area or several. It will depend on the area of study, so in the case of a small joint effusion will be only on one area, in the case of muscles it is advisable to perform in its proximal, middle, and distal third.

6. It is necessary to know the indications prior to the study; for example, in the case of a muscular study, it is required to know if the patient must remain at rest and if so, for how long, or if the study can be performed with flexion or extension in the case of the extremities. SWE measures must, in practice, be taken from a patient who is completely still.

7. Finally, it is recommended that in the case of periodical controls of the stiffness values obtained, these should always be carried out with the same equipment.

1.6 Shear Wave Elastography: Artefacts in Muscles and Tendons

1.6.1 Signal Void Area

2D-SWE elastograms may present areas without any information on the medium. These areas, considered null values, are not coded on the colour map, and appear in black. This is referred to as a "*signal void area*" (Fig. 1.24).

Bouchet [51] gives a complete description of the causes that can generate it:

- Incorrect acquisition settings in B-mode ultrasound and SWE mode
- Existence of liquid
- Posterior elastographic shadowing artefact
- Lesion too stiff
- Intralesional necrosis
- Lesion too hypoechoic
- Depth of analysis is too great

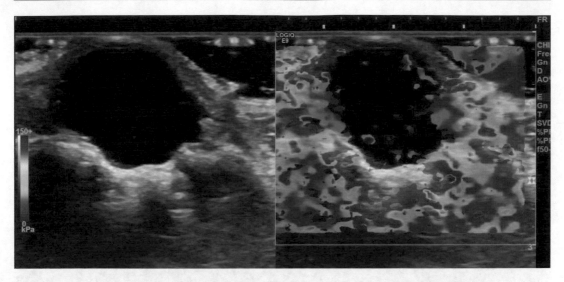

Fig. 1.24 "Signal void area"

Fig. 1.25 "Black Hole Phenomenon"

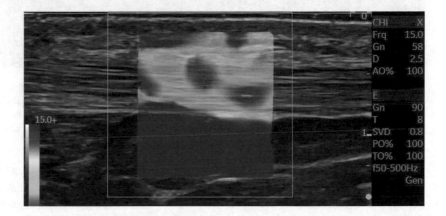

1.6.2 Black Hole Phenomenon

When the medium is too stiff, it is not possible to track shear wave propagation even with an ultra-fast frame rate. As a result, SWE elasticity values are considered null (Fig. 1.25).

1.6.3 Pseudo-Liquid Lesions

In 2D-SWE, signal void areas may also mean that the device did not detect any speckle movement when shear waves pass over because of a highly hypoechoic environment.

For example, myxoid lesions appear as pseudo-liquid lesions in standard B-mode and

SWE mode, whereas they are solid and vascularized in Doppler mode [50].

1.6.4 Musculotendinous Anisotropy

Muscles and tendons combine some elastic properties of solids, viscous properties of liquids, and properties related to their anisotropy. Because of this, calculating Young's modulus involves a complex transversally isotropic rheological model not yet used in common practice [52]. Anisotropy of muscles or tendons should not be considered an artefact, but rather an inherent characteristic of these structures.

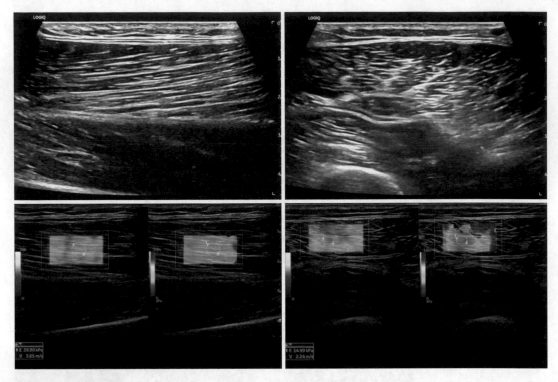

Fig. 1.26 The shear modulus is influenced by the probe's orientation about the structures being studied, and SWE is sensitive to transducer pressure and angle. The anisotropy of muscles and tendons determines that the elastographic study of these structures must be done in a very proto-colized way. It is only parallel to the fibre axis that mechanical properties of anisotropic mediums can be directly calculated from the shear wave velocity

The importance of the angulation of the probe relative to the muscle fibre axis in the quantization of the results has been demonstrated [53].

When measurements are made parallel to the fibre axis rather than perpendicularly, shear wave velocities within anisotropic materials like striated muscle, and tendons are significantly higher [52].

1.6.5 Only Elasticity Measurements Measured Perpendicular to the Fibre Axis Are Representative of the Medium's Mechanical Properties

Orientation of the muscle fibres affects shear wavefront attenuation. When the wavefront is perpendicular to the fibre axis, it is substantial but negligible when the wavefront is parallel. Muscle and tendon are transversely isotropic. It is only parallel to the fibre axis that mechanical properties of anisotropic mediums are consistent with Voigt's model underlying SWE physical principles, and that Young's modulus can be directly calculated from the shear wave velocity (Fig. 1.26).

The shear modulus is influenced by the probe's orientation about the structures being studied, and SWE is sensitive to transducer pressure and angle and for that reason, light pressure with the transducer is recommended [4, 10].

For the calculation of the elastograms, most US elastography equipment demands a minimum distance (often 1–2 mm) between the structure of interest and the skin's surface. The usage of gel spacers to satisfy this criterion, because slim people may not be able to see this minimum distance, has not been proved to accurately generate the same outcomes.

Poor contact and coupling between the probe and tissue can prevent the energy of the push

Fig. 1.27 SWE study of Achilles tendon shows that poor contact and coupling between the probe and tissue can prevent the energy of the push pulse from being transmitted into the tissue

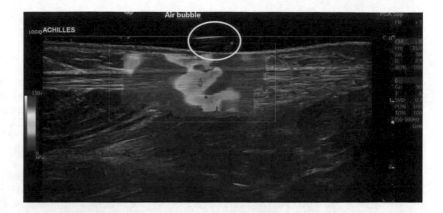

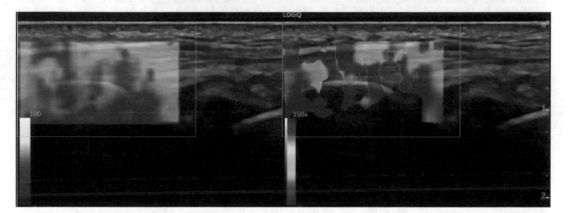

Fig. 1.28 Artefact secondary to reverberation echoes from *a strong reflector-like bone*

pulse from being transmitted into the tissue. This results in low shear wave amplitude which can cause inaccurate shear wave measurements and poor color fill (Fig. 1.27).

1.6.6   Reverberation Echoes from a Strong Reflector-Like Bone Can Cause Artefacts in Shear Wave Elastography (Fig. 1.28)

The assessment of the stiffness of certain tendon structures such as the Achilles tendon or the supraspinatus or infraspinatus tendons can be affected by the reverberation artefact created by adjacent bone surfaces.

Nowadays, the increased power of the new probes can reduce this artefact.

References

1. Lavarello R, Oelze ML. Theory of ultrasound physics and imaging. In: Ultrasound elastography for biomedical applications and medicine. Hoboken: Wiley; 2019. ISBN 9781119021551.
2. Nenadic I, Urban M, Greenleaf J, Gennisson J-L, Bernal M, Tanter M. Editors' introduction. In: Ultrasound elastography for biomedical applications and medicine. Hoboken: Wiley; 2019. ISBN 9781119021551.
3. Ormachea J, Parker KJ. Elastography imaging: the 30-year perspective. Phys Med Biol. 2020;65(24) https://doi.org/10.1088/1361-6560/abca00.
4. Prado-Costa R, Rebelo J, Monteiro-Barroso J, Preto AS. Ultrasound elastography: compression elastography and shear-wave elastography in the assessment of tendon injury. Insights Imaging. 2018;9(5):791–814. https://doi.org/10.1007/s13244-018-0642-1. Epub 2018 Aug 17.
5. Gunnison J-L. Transverse wave propagation in anisotropic media. In: Ultrasound elastography for biomedical applications and medicine. Hoboken: Wiley; 2019. ISBN 9781119021551.

6. Vasconcelos L, Gennisson J-L, Nenadic I. Continuum mechanics tensor calculus and solutions to wave equations. In: Ultrasound elastography for biomedical applications and medicine. Hoboken: Wiley; 2019. ISBN 9781119021551.

7. https://en.wikipedia.org/wiki/Constitutive_equation.

8. https://en.wikipedia.org/wiki/Poisson%27s_ratio.

9. Wang M. Ultrasound tomography. In: Industrial tomography systems and applications, Woodhead publishing series in electronic and optical materials. Cambridge: Woodhead Publishing; 2015. p. 235–61.

10. Taljanovic MS, Gimber LH, Becker GW, Latt LD, Klauser AS, Melville DM, Gao L, Witte RS. Shear-wave elastography: basic physics and musculoskeletal applications. Radiographics. 2017;37(3):855–70. https://doi.org/10.1148/rg.2017160116.

11. Budday S, Ovaert TC, Holzapfel GA, et al. Fifty shades of brain: a review on the mechanical testing and modeling of brain tissue. Arch Computat Methods Eng. 2020;27:1187–230. https://doi.org/10.1007/s11831-019-09352-w.

12. Wang Y, Insana MF. Wave propagation in viscoelastic materials. In: Ultrasound elastography for biomedical applications and medicine. Hoboken: Wiley; 2019. ISBN 9781119021551.

13. Sigrist RMS, Liau J, Kaffas AE, Chammas MC, Willmann JK. Ultrasound elastography: review of techniques and clinical applications. Theranostics. 2017;7(5):1303–29. https://doi.org/10.7150/thno.18650.

14. https://en.wikipedia.org/wiki/Continuum_mechanics.

15. Chen W. The renaissance of continuum mechanics. J Zheijang Univ-Sci. 2014;15:231–40. https://doi.org/10.1631/jzus.A1400079.

16. Liu I-S, Sampaio R. On objectivity and the principle of material frame-indifference. Mecánica Computacional. XXXI:1553–69.

17. Li GY, Cao Y. Mechanics of ultrasound elastography. Proc Math Phys Eng Sci. 2017 Mar;473(2199):20160841 https://doi.org/10.1098/rspa.2016.0841. Epub 2017 Mar 1.

18. Lerner RM, Parker KJ, Holen J, Gramiak R, Waag RC. Sonoelasticity: Medical elasticity images derived from ultrasound signals in mechanically vibrated targets. Acoust Imaging 1988;16:317–27.

19. Parker KJ, Fu D, Graceswki SM, Yeung F, Levinson SF. Vibration sonoelastography and the detectability of lesions. Ultrasound Med Biol. 1998;24(9):1437–47. https://doi.org/10.1016/s0301-5629(98)00123-9.

20. Dawood M, Ibrahim N, Elsaeed H, Hegazy N Diagnostic performance of sonoelastographic Tsukuba score and strain ratio in evaluation of breast masses. The Egyptian Journal of Radiology and Nuclear Medicine. 2018;49(01):265–71.

21. Wadugodapitiya S, Sakamoto M, Sugita K, Morise Y, Tanaka M, Kobayashi K. Ultrasound elastographic assessment of the stiffness of the anteromedial knee joint capsule at varying knee angles. Biomed Mater Eng. 2019;30(2):219–30. https://doi.org/10.3233/BME-191046.

22. Patra S, Grover SB. Physical principles of elastography: a primer for radiologists. Indographics. 2022;1:27–40. 10.1055/s-0042-1742575

23. Dewall RJ. Ultrasound elastography: principles, techniques, and clinical applications. Crit Rev Biomed Eng. 2013;41(1):1–19. https://doi.org/10.1615/critrevbiomedeng.2013006991.

24. Czernuszewicz TJ, Gallippi CM. Acoustic radiation force impulse ultrasound. In: Ultrasound elastography for biomedical applications and medicine. Hoboken: Wiley; 2019. ISBN 9781119021551.

25. Gennisson J-L, Tanter M. Supersonic shear imaging. In: Ultrasound elastography for biomedical applications and medicine. Hoboken: Wiley; 2019. ISBN 9781119021551.

26. Sandrin L, Sasso M, Audière S, Bastard C, Fournier C, Oudry J, Miette V, Catheline S. Transient elastography: from research to noninvasive assessment of liver fibrosis using Fibroscan®. In: Ultrasound elastography for biomedical applications and medicine. Hoboken: Wiley; 2019. ISBN 9781119021551.

27. User manual of Fibroscan® 630 Europe.

28. McAleavey SA. Single tracking location shear wave elastography. In: Ultrasound elastography for biomedical applications and medicine. Hoboken: Wiley; 2019. ISBN 9781119021551.

29. Lu J, Chen M, Chen Q-H, Wu Q, Jiang J-N, Leung T-Y. Elastogram: physics, clinical applications, and risks. Maternal-Fetal Med. 2019;1(2):113–22. https://doi.org/10.1097/FM9.0000000000000024.

30. Alizad A, Fatemi M. Vibro-acoustography and its medical applications. In: Ultrasound elastography for biomedical applications and medicine. Hoboken: Wiley; 2019. ISBN 9781119021551.

31. Gennisson JL, Deffieux T, Fink M, Tanter M. Ultrasound elastography: principles and techniques. Diagn Interv Imaging. 2013;94(5):487–95. https://doi.org/10.1016/j.diii.2013.01.022. Epub 2013 Apr 22.

32. Konofagou E. Harmonic motion imaging. In: Ultrasound elastography for biomedical applications and medicine. Hoboken: Wiley; 2019. ISBN 9781119021551.

33. Vappou J, Maleke C, Konofagou EE. Quantitative viscoelastic parameters measured by harmonic motion imaging. Phys Med Biol. 2009;54(11):3579–94.

34. Konofagou EE, Maleke C, Vappou J. Harmonic motion imaging (HMI) for tumor imaging and treatment monitoring. Curr Med Imaging Rev. 2012;8(1):16–26.

35. McAleavey S, Collins E, Kelly J, et al. Validation of SMURF estimation of shear modulus in hydrogels. Ultrason Imaging. 2009;31:131–50.

36. Song P, Chen S. Comb-push ultrasound shear elastography. In: Ultrasound elastography for biomedical applications and medicine. Hoboken: Wiley; 2019. ISBN 9781119021551.

37. Song P, Manduca A, Zhao H, et al. Fast shear compounding using robust 2-D shear wave speed calculation and multi-directional filtering. Ultrasound Med Biol. 2014;40:1343–55.

38. Song, P. (2014). Innovations in ultrasound shear wave elastography. PhD Thesis. Department of Physiology and Biomedical Engineering, Mayo Clinic College of Medicine, Rochester, USA.

39. Mahdavi SS, Moradi M, Wen X, Morris WJ, Salcudean SE. Vibro-elastography for visualization of the prostate region: method evaluation. Med Image Comput Comput Assist Interv. 2009;12(Pt 2):339–47. https://doi.org/10.1007/978-3-642-04271-3_42.

40. Zhang X, Zhou B, VanBuren WM, Burnett TL, Knudsen JM. Transvaginal ultrasound vibro-elastography for measuring uterine viscoelasticity: a phantom study. Ultrasound Med Biol. 2019;45(2):617–22. https://doi.org/10.1016/j.ultrasmedbio.2018.10.009. Epub 2018 Nov 19.

41. Wu Z, Taylor LS, Rubens DJ, Parker KJ. Sonoelastographic imaging of interference patterns for estimation of the shear velocity of homogeneous biomaterials. Phys Med Biol. 2004;49:911–22.

42. Hoyt K, Castaneda B, Parker KJ. Two-dimensional sonoelastographic shear velocity imaging. Ultrasound Med Biol. 2008;34:276–88.

43. Parker KJ. Dynamic elasticity imaging. In: Ultrasound elastography for biomedical applications and medicine. Hoboken: Wiley; 2019. ISBN 9781119021551.

44. Tzschatzsch H, Ipek-Ugay S, Trong MN, Guo J, Eggers J, Gentz E, Fischer T, Schultz M, Braun J, Sack I. Multifrequency time-harmonic elastography for the measurement of liver viscoelasticity in large tissue windows. Ultrasound Med Biol. 2015;41:724–33.

45. Tzschatzsch H, Nguyen Trong M, Scheuermann T, Ipek-Ugay S, Fischer T, Schultz M, Braun J, Sack I. Two-dimensional time-harmonic elastography of the human liver and spleen. Ultrasound Med Biol. 2016;42:2562–7.

46. Parker KJ, Ormachea J, Zvietcovich F, Castaneda B. Reverberant shear wave fields and estimation of tissue properties. Phys Med Biol. 2017;62:1046–61.

47. Ormachea J, Parker KJ, Barr RG. An initial study of complete 2D shear wave dispersion images using a reverberant shear wave field. Phys Med Biol. 2019;64:145009.

48. Dietrich CF, Bamber J, Berzigotti A, et al. EFSUMB guidelines and recommendations on the clinical use of liver ultrasound elastography, update 2017 (long version). Ultraschall Med. 2017;38:e16–47.

49. Ormachea J, Zvietcovich F. Reverberant shear wave elastography: a multi-modal and multi-scale approach to measure the viscoelasticity properties of soft tissues. Front Phys. 2020; https://doi.org/10.3389/fphy.2020.606793.

50. Bamber J, Cosgrove D, Dietrich CF, et al. EFSUMB guidelines and recommendations on the clinical use of ultrasound elastography, part 1: basic principles and technology. Ultraschall Med. 2013;34:169–84.

51. Kot BCW, Zhang ZJ, Lee AWC, et al. Elastic modulus of muscle and tendon with shear wave ultrasound elastography: variations with different technical settings. PLoS One. 2012;7:e44348.

52. Bouchet P, Gennisson JL, Podda A, Alilet M, Carrié M, Aubry S. Artifacts and technical restrictions in 2D shear wave elastography. Ultraschall Med. 2020;41(3):267–77. https://doi.org/10.1055/a-0805-1099.

53. Aubry S, Nueffer JP, Carrié M. Evaluation of the effect of an anisotropic medium on shear wave velocities of intra-muscular gelatinous inclusions. Ultrasound Med Biol. 2017;43(1):301–8. https://doi.org/10.1016/j.ultrasmedbio.2016.09.006. Epub 2016 Oct 12.

Skin and Soft Parts Benign Pathology

2

Fernando Alfageme Roldán

2.1 Introduction

Since Hippocratic medicine, palpation has played an important role in the general physical examination of patients because it provides information about the physical characteristics of the tissues [1]. A loss of elasticity or increase in rigidity of organs or tissues has traditionally been associated with a poorer prognosis in inflammatory processes, which histologically tend to be associated with fibrosis, and in tumor processes, in which the elastic properties of healthy tissues decrease [2, 3].

Estimation of the elasticity or rigidity of tissues could therefore facilitate early, noninvasive monitoring and treatment of inflammatory and tumor processes [4].

Elastography is a technique in which ultrasound is used to detect changes in the elasticity of tissues [5]. Since the late twentieth century, elastography has been used in various diseases, including tumors of the breast, thyroid, and liver, as well as in inflammatory processes in the same organs [6].

The recent introduction of high-frequency linear ultrasound probes has made it possible for this technology to be applied to superficial tissues such as the bone and muscle system [6], and the skin [7].

It is important to note that most cutaneous elastography studies are small case series, a majority of which are observational and of limited scientific robustness.

Nevertheless, the possibilities of this technique to assess the features of skin tissues added to B and color Doppler findings, completes a multimodal ultrasound skin evaluation.

2.1.1 Elastography: The Physical Concepts of Strain and Shear Wave

When a tissue is subjected to pressure, it deforms and tends to recover its initial shape (elasticity). The resistance of the tissue to deformation is called rigidity or stiffness [8, 9].

The term strain describes the change in the relative length of a structure subjected to pressure with respect to the surrounding tissue (Fig. 2.1).

In addition to this physical phenomenon, a series of waves perpendicular to the displacement of the pressure wave, known as shear waves, are also generated in the tissue [10]. It is possible to determine the velocity of the shear wave, which provides indirect quantitative information about the stiffness of the tissue.

F. Alfageme Roldán (✉)
Dermatologic Department, Hospital Universitario
Puerta de Hierro Majadahonda, Madrid, Spain

Fig. 2.1 When a tissue is compressed with a force F, its particles (A) undergo a displacement (A'). The quotient between the displacement of the structure under study (*d*) and the initial total length *D* is called strain. Perpendicular to this pressure wave there is a displacement of the particles that generate waves called shear waves

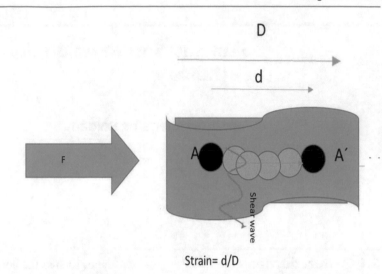

Strain= d/D

2.1.2 Types of Elastography and their Limitations

According to the clinical guidelines on elastography published by the European Federation of Societies for Ultrasound in Medicine and Biology (EFSUMB) [11] there are two basic types of elastography: strain elastography (SE), which assesses tissue deformation, and shear wave elastography (SWE), which characterizes the shear waves.

Elastography can also be classified according to the physical force that produces the tissue deformation. This force can be mechanical (manual or automatic) or it can be produced by an ultrasound pulse called acoustic radiation force impulse (ARFI). Each of these elastography methods offers qualitative or quantitative information about the rigidity or stiffness (terms used interchangeably in this review) of tissues.

Semiquantitative measurement scales normally associate a number from 1 to 5 with the rigidity percentage of a structure, with 1 being softest and 5 being stiffest [11].

Another way to quantify the stiffness of a structure is to express it in relation to the surrounding parenchyma. This quotient is known as the strain ratio [12].

In SWE, which determines shear wave displacement velocities, measurements are quantitative and can be expressed in either kPa or m/s [13].

Inter- and intraobserver variability is greater in SE (especially the manual variant) than in SWE [11].

However, as in the case of conventional ultrasound, these artifacts also provide information about the structure being examined [14].

2.2 Elastography in Dermatology: Technique and Peculiarities

According to the EFSUMB clinical guidelines on elastography [11], the following recommendations should be considered when elastography is performed on any organ:

1. The structure should be in close proximity to the transducer (<4 cm).
2. The structure should be nearly homogeneous.
3. When pressure is applied, there should be no slippage in the structure over deeper planes.
4. Pressure should be applied by a surface larger than the structure being examined.
5. No structures that damp compression, such as large blood vessels, should be present.
6. The structures being examined should be completely included within the region of interest.

7. The direction of the compression force should be known.
8. The number of structures being examined should be limited.

When elastography is used on the skin, gel should not be used in the region of interest [11]. As we can infer, the skin is an organ that adapts to the conditions in which elastography can be carried out with the appropriate technique and technology, that is, high-frequency linear probes applied to the skin and adnexa [15].

2.3   Elastography of Normal Skin and Adnexa

The stiffness of healthy skin varies according to the cutaneous layer being studied. The dermis is more rigid than the subcutaneous cellular tissue [16] (Fig. 2.2).

In the subcutaneous cellular tissue, the septa are more rigid than the fat lobules. Blood vessels, like the peripheral nerves, are not very rigid in comparison to the surrounding subcutaneous cellular tissue [16]. Regarding nail elastography nail plate is harder than the nail bed (Fig. 2.3).

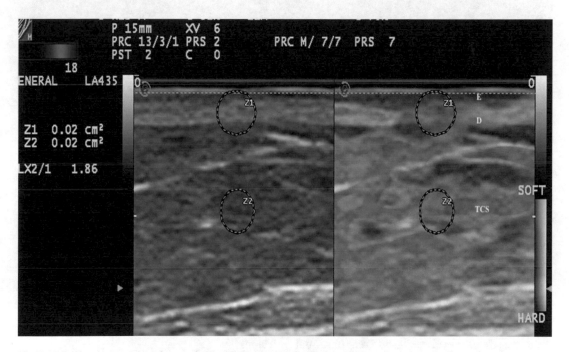

Fig. 2.2 Strain elastography of normal skin (E. Epidermis, D, dermis, TCS, subcutaneous cellular tissue). Note the stiffness ratio of dermis and fat SR = 1.86 indicating that the dermis is stiffer than the subcutaneous cellular tissue

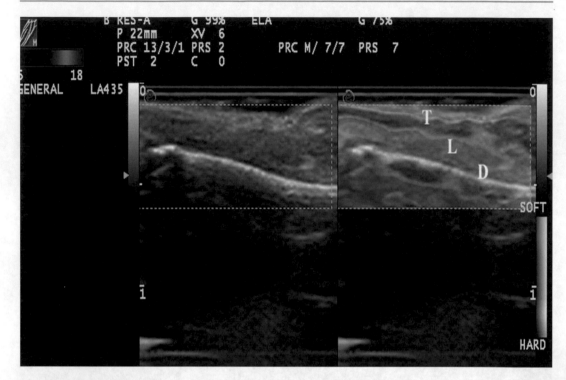

Fig. 2.3 Nail strain elastography. The nail plate (T) is harder than the bed (L) and similar to the distal phalanx (F)

2.4 Benign Skin Tumors and Neck Masses

Although benign subcutaneous tumors have a recognizable appearance in B-mode ultrasound [17] in doubtful cases elastography could play a useful role in the differential diagnosis.

In a study by Bhatia et al. [18], 52 non-nodal neck masses were evaluated using real-time qualitative ultrasound elastography.

The diagnosis of the lesions was later corroborated by cytology and histology. The lesions were evaluated semiquantitatively on a scale of 0–3, where 0 was completely soft and 3 was completely stiff.

Lipomas were less stiff than other types of lesions, most of which were cysts, malformations, and neurogenic tumors (Fig. 2.4).

In an extension of the study [19], SWE was used to assess malignant and benign neck tumors. The mean stiffness of the malignant tumors (226.4 kPa) was higher than that of the benign lesions (28.3 kPa) and the difference was statistically significant

With a cut-off of 174.4 kPa, sensitivity of 83.3% and specificity of 97.5% were achieved in the differentiation of benign and malignant lesions.

The authors noted that all tumors were correctly diagnosed with conventional ultrasound and that elastography would not have altered the treatment, but they argued that less experienced operators could find the technique helpful in the diagnosis of neck lesions.

Park et al. [20] used elastography to differentiate inflamed and unruptured epidermal cysts, the latter being stiffer than the former (Fig. 2.4b).

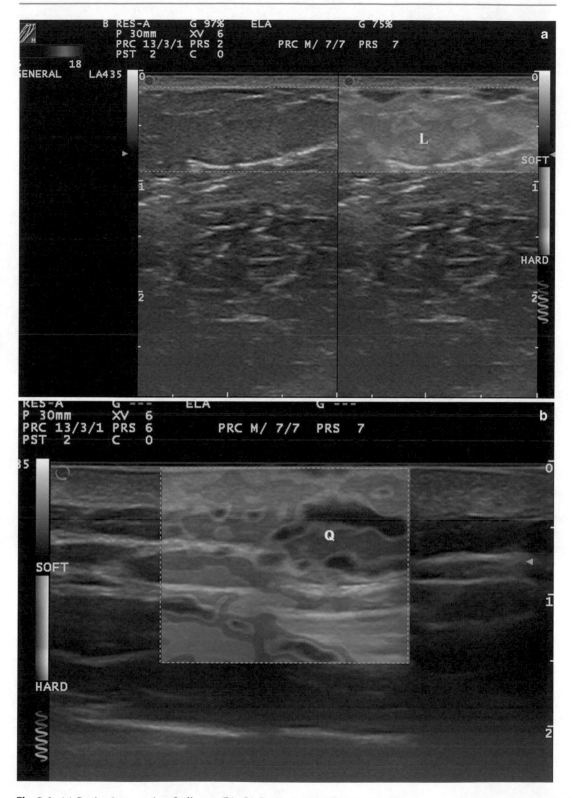

Fig. 2.4 (a) Strain elastography of a lipoma (L). (b) Strain elastography of a cyst (Q)

2.5   Malignant Skin Tumors

Elastography shows that malignant skin tumors are stiffer than the surrounding tissue (Fig. 2.5).

Dasgeb et al. [21] studied 55 patients with a total of 67 epithelial tumors, of which 29 were malignant (17 basal cell carcinomas and 12 squamous cell carcinomas) and 19 were benign. In this study, the strain ratio was >3.9 in all malignant skin tumors and <3 in all benign skin tumors.

For strain ratio values between 3.00 and 3.9, sensitivity and specificity were 100% in the diagnosis of malignant lesions.

Elastography has been used to study melanoma.

In a pilot study by Botar et al. [22] 42 melanomas in 39 patients were studied using SE and color Doppler ultrasound to assess vascularization.

The use of elastography in the evaluation of biologic behavior of basal cell carcinomas, some authors like Liang et al., indicate that high-risk basal cell carcinoma are harder than low-risk BCC [23]. Our group also published a paper on the increased marginal strain of infiltrative BCC vs non-infiltrative BCC [24].

The correlation between melanoma neovascularization and prognosis is well known in the literature [25]. This correlation with lesions together with stiffness could be a prognostic factor in melanoma [26].

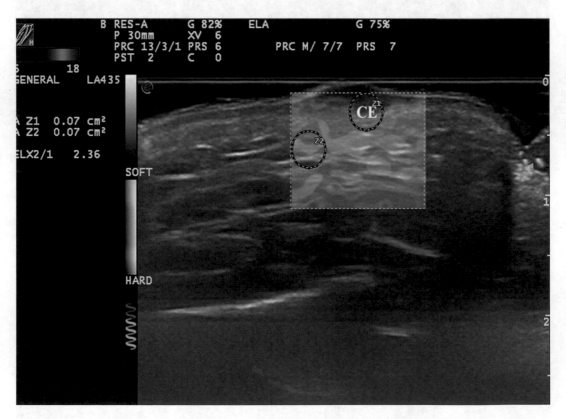

Fig. 2.5 Strain elastography in epidermoid carcinoma of the cheek (CE). SR = 2.36 indicates that it is harder than the adjacent subcutaneous cellular tissue

2.6   Lymph Node Enlargement

The aim of ultrasound assessment of lymph nodes is to noninvasively diagnose malignant lymph nodes in patients with clinically suspicious lesions [27, 28].

Lymph nodes have an elastic structure in which the cortex tends to be less rigid than the capsule and the hilum (Fig. 2.6).

To assess the stiffness of lymph nodes, SE is used to classify nodes into 4 or 5 categories according to the proportion of stiff areas they present [28].

Benign enlarged nodes generally tend to be soft, whereas malignant nodes tend to be stiffer [29].

However, lymphomas are less stiff than metastatic nodes and similar in stiffness to inflamed nodes. Therefore, benign and lymphomatous nodes cannot be distinguished with elastography alone [30].

In the case of melanoma, Hinz et al. [31] found that elastography in addition to conventional B-mode sonography combined with color Doppler sonography increased sensitivity in the detection of metastatic disease (Fig. 2.7) in clinically suspicious enlarged lymph but found no increase in specificity (76.2%). Similar results were obtained in later studies such as that of Ogata et al. [32] (Fig. 2.7).

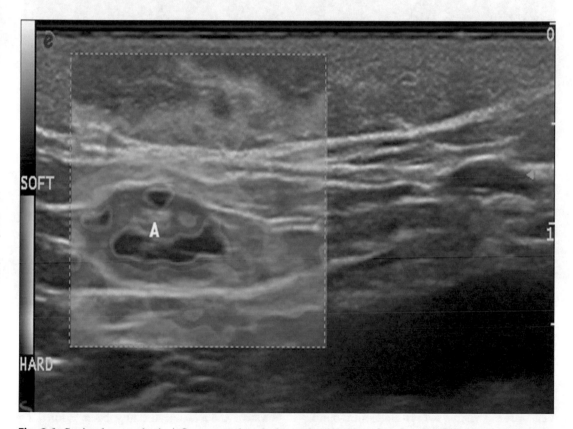

Fig. 2.6 Strain elastography in inflammatory lymphadenopathy (A). Note that the medullary is harder than the cortical

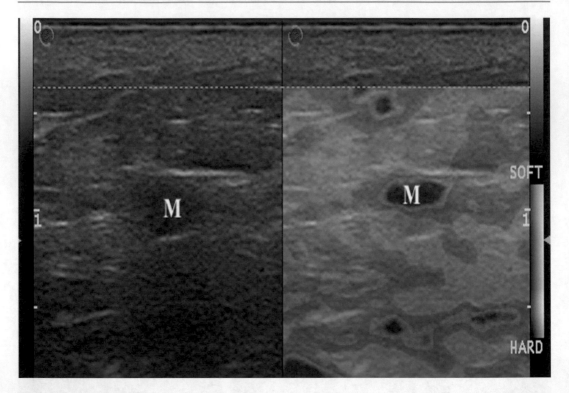

Fig. 2.7 Strain elastography in a melanoma lymph node metastasis (M), note the complete stiffness of the lesion without soft zones

2.7 Elastography in Inflammatory Skin Diseases

Inflammation not only causes changes in the sonographic structure of the skin and adnexa in B-mode and Doppler ultrasound [33] it also affects the stiffness of the structures.

In a study by Gaspari et al. [34], 50 patients who visited the emergency department for abscess drainage were examined using B-mode ultrasound and SE. With elastography, it was possible to observe stiff areas around the abscesses that were not visible with B-mode ultrasound.

Cucos et al. [35] measured the effects of topical corticosteroid treatment on epidermal and dermal thickness and elasticity in 16 psoriatic plaques. Epidermal thickness decreased, whereas dermal thickness increased slightly and there was no change in plaque elasticity.

Despite the small number of patients in this study, the results seem to indicate that the sensitivity of SE in the treatment of psoriatic plaques is low.

In a recent paper, using SW elastography, Guazzaroni et al. [36] in a series of 26 patients found a reduction in stiffness and vascularization of responsive psoriatic plaques.

Asil et al. [37] found increased strain in psoriatic nails compared with control nails. This increase in nail strain correlated with NAPSI scores.

The use of elastography in hidradenitis suppurativa tunnels has recently been studied by Iznardo et al. as a tool to evaluate fibrosis in these structures [38].

Elastography has been more extensively developed in fibrotic and sclerotic processes that are primarily cutaneous or systemic (morphea/systemic sclerosis), in which clinical measure-

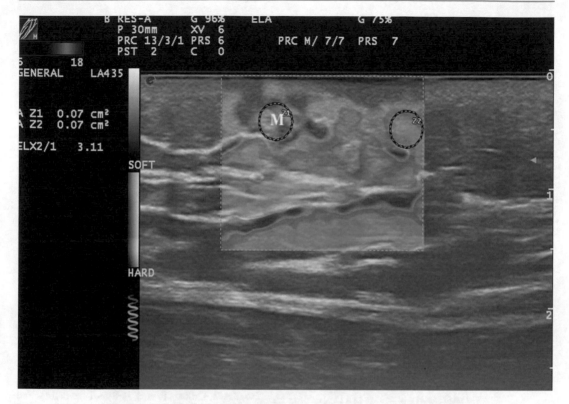

Fig. 2.8 Elastography in morphea (M). Increased hardness of the dermo-subdermal interface can be seen in the plaque with respect to the surrounding tissue (SR = 3.4)

ment scales have very limited sensitivity and specificity [39] (Fig. 2.8).

Initial studies carried out with SE in systemic sclerosis, such as that of Iagnocco et al. [39] have indicated that dermal stiffness is greater in patients with systemic sclerosis than in controls. However, the reproducibility of the technique at other sites, such as the fingers, was variable, perhaps because of the proximity of the bony surface of the phalanges.

Di Geso et al. [40] repeated this exercise to determine the degree of correlation between measurements with SE and with B-mode ultrasound. The authors concluded that elastography reduces inter- and intraobserver variability in the assessment of dermal thickness of the fingers in patients with systemic sclerosis.

Tumsatan et al. [41] compared a cohort of 29 patients with systemic sclerosis and 29 controls and found significative increased hardness in the skin of these patients, with a good correlation with clinical palpation scores.

2.8 Elastography in Other Skin Diseases

Recently in the field of alopecias, some groups have explored the possibility of assessment of fibrotic tissue through SWE in scarring alopecias [41] and even in patients with pre-androgenetic alopecias in which early loss of rigidity and thinning of dermis and subcutaneous tissue may predict this type of hair loss pattern [42].

2.9 Clinical Applications

A summary of the findings in different clinical conditions can be found in Table 2.1.

Table 2.1 A summary of the findings in different clinical conditions

Application in dermatologic ultrasound	Findings and confirmation in shear wave (SW) and strain elastography (SE)	References
Benign tumors Cysts, lipomas	Benign lesions tend to be softer than malignant lesions (SW) (SE)	Bhatia et al. [18]
Basal cell carcinoma (BCC)	BCC tends to be stiffer and more aggressive variants are stiffer (SW) (SE)	Liang et al. [23] Alfageme et al. [24]
Melanoma	Melanomas are stiffer than benign melanocytic lesions (SE)	Hinz et al. [26]
Psoriasis	Psoriatic plaque is stiffer than the surrounding skin (SW)	Guazzaroni et al. [36]
Hidradenitis suppurativa	Tunnels are stiffer than surrounding tissue (SW)	Iznardo et al. [38]
Systemic sclerosis	Sclerotic skin is stiffer in patients with systemic sclerosis/morphea (SE) (SW)	Iagnocco et al. [39] Di Geso et al. [40]

2.10 Conclusion and Future Perspectives

Elastography in dermatology is an emerging technique with great potential in the physical characterization of the tissues of the skin and adnexa. The various elastography techniques offer complementary and synergistic information in the assessment of cutaneous tissues. Dermatologists can consider scenarios in which elastography can offer complementary information that would improve patient care.

References

1. Alix-Panabieres C, Magliocco A, Cortes-Hernandez LE, Eslami-S Z, Franklin D, Messina JL. Detection of cancer metastasis: past, present and future. Clin Exp Metastasis. 2022;39(1):21–8.
2. Egeblad M, Rasch M, Weaver V. Dynamic interplay between the collagen scaffold and tumor evolution. Curr Opin Cell Biol. 2010;22:697–706.
3. Huang S, Ingber DE. Cell tension, matrix mechanics, and cancer development. Cancer Cell. 2005;8:175–6.
4. Oberai A, Gokhale N, Goenezen S, Barbone P, Hall T, Sommer A, et al. Linear and nonlinear elasticity imaging of soft tissue in vivo: demonstration of feasibility. Phys Med Biol. 2009;54:1191–207.
5. Garra B. Imaging and estimation of tissue elasticity by ultrasound. Ultrasound Q. 2007;23:255–68.
6. Cosgrove D, Piscaglia F, Bamber J, Bojunga J, Correas J, Gilja O, et al. EFSUMB guidelines and recommendations on the clinical use of ultrasound elastography. Part 2: clinical applications. Ultraschall Med. 2013;34:238–53.
7. Alfageme F, Cerezo E, Roustan G. Real-time elastography in inflammatory skin diseases: a Primer. Ultrasound Medi Biol. 2015;41:S82–3.
8. Wells P, Liang H. Medical ultrasound: imaging of soft tissue strain and elasticity. J R Soc Interface. 2011;8:1521–49.
9. Housden R, Chen L, Gee A, Treece G, Uff C, Fromageau J, et al. A new method for the acquisition of ultrasonic strain image volumes. Ultrasound Med Biol. 2011;37:434–41.
10. Sarvazyan A, Rudenko O, Swanson S, Fowlkes J, Emelianov S. Shear wave elasticity imaging: A new ultrasonic technology of medical diagnostics. Ultrasound Med Biol. 1998;24:1419–35.
11. Bamber J, Cosgrove D, Dietrich CF, Fromageau J, Bojunga J, Calliada F, et al. EFSUMB guidelines and recommendations on the clinical use of ultrasound elastography. Part 1: basic principles and technology. Ultraschall Med. 2013;34:169–84.
12. Havre R, Waage J, Gilja O, Odegaard S, Nesje L. Realtime elastography: Strain ratio measurements are influenced by the position of the reference area. Ultraschall Med. 2012;33:559–68.
13. Palmeri M, Nightingale R. Acoustic radiation force-based elasticity imaging methods. Interface Focus. 2011;1:553–64.
14. Thitaikumar A, Ophir J. Effect of lesion boundary conditions on axial strain elastograms: a parametric study. Ultrasound Med Biol. 2007;33:1463–7.
15. Coutts L, Miller N, Harland C, Bamber J. Feasibility of skin surface elastography by tracking skin surface topography. J Biomed Opt. 2013;18:121513.
16. Osanai O, Ohtsuka M, Hotta M, Kitaharai T, Takema Y. A new method for the visualization and quantification of internal skin elasticity by ultrasound imaging. Skin Res Technol. 2011;17:270–7.
17. Wortsman X. Sonography of the nail. In: Wortsman X, Jemec GBE, editors. Dermatologic ultrasound with clinical and histological correlation. New York: Springer; 2013. p. 421.
18. Bhatia K, Rasalkar D, Lee Y, Wong K, King A, Yuen Y, et al. Real-time qualitative ultrasound elastography of miscellaneous non-nodal neck masses: applications and limitations. Ultrasound Med Biol. 2010;36:1644–52.
19. Bhatia K, Yuen E, Cho C, Tong C, Lee Y, Ahuja A. A pilot study evaluating real-time shear wave ultrasound elastography of miscellaneous non-nodal neck

masses in a routine head and neck ultrasound clinic. Ultrasound Med Biol. 2012;38:933–42.

20. Park J, Chae I, Kwon D. Utility of sonoelastography in differentiating ruptured from unruptured epidermal cysts and implications for patient care. J Ultrasound Med. 2015;34:1175–81.

21. Dasgeb B, Morris MA, Mehregan D, Siegel EL. Quantified ultrasound elastography in the assessment of cutaneous carcinoma. Br J Radiol. 2015;88:2015034.

22. Botar C, Bolboaca S, Cosgarea R, Şenilă S, Rogojan L, Lenghel M, et al. Doppler ultrasound and strain elastography in the assessment of cutaneous melanoma: preliminary results. Med Ultrason. 2015;17:509–14.

23. Liang JF, Feng MC, Luo PP, Guan JY, Chen GF, Wu SY, Wang J, Feng MY. High-frequency ultrasound and shear wave elastography in quantitative differential diagnosis of high-risk and low-risk basal cell carcinomas. J Ultrasound Med. 2022;41:1447–54.

24. Alfageme F, Salgüero I, Nájera L, Suarez ML, Roustan G. Increased marginal stiffness differentiates infiltrative from noninfiltrative cutaneous basal cell carcinomas in the facial area: a prospective study. J Ultrasound Med. 2019;38:1841–5.

25. Lassau N, Lamuraglia M, Koscielny S, Spatz A, Roche A, Leclere J, et al. Prognostic value of angiogenesis evaluated with high frequency and colour Doppler sonography for preoperative assessment of primary cutaneous melanomas: correlation with recurrence after a 5 year follow-up period. Cancer Imaging. 2006;6(1):24–9.

26. Hinz T, Wenzel J, Schmid-Wendtner M. Real-time tissue elastography: a helpful tool in the diagnosis of cutaneous melanoma? J Am Acad Dermatol. 2011;65:424–6.

27. Choi Y, Lee J, Baek J. Ultrasound elastography for evaluation of cervical lymph nodes. Ultrasonography. 2015;34:157–64.

28. Tan R, Xiao Y, He Q. Ultrasound elastography: its potential role in assessment of cervical lymphadenopathy. Acad Radiol. 2010;17:849.

29. Alam F, Naito K, Horiguchi J, Fukuda H, Tachikake T, Ito K. Accuracy of sonographic elastography in the differential diagnosis of enlarged cervical lymph nodes: comparison with conventional B-mode sonography. AJR Am J Roentgenol. 2008;191:604.

30. Bhatia K, Cho C, Tong C, Yuen E, Ahuja A. Shear wave elasticity imaging of cervical lymph nodes. Ultrasound Med Biol. 2012;38:195–201.

31. Hinz T, Hoeller T, Wenzel J, Bieber T, Schmid-Wendtner M. Real-time tissue elastography as promising diagnostic tool for diagnosis of lymph node

metastases in patients with malignant melanoma: a prospective single-center experience. Dermatology. 2013;226:81–90.

32. Ogata D, Uematsu T, Yoshikawa S, Kiyohara Y. Accuracy of realtime ultrasound elastography in the differential diagnosis of lymph nodes in cutaneous malignant melanoma (CMM): a pilot study. Int J Clin Oncol. 2014;19:716–21.

33. Echeverría-García B, Borbujo J, Alfageme F. The use of ultrasound imaging in dermatology. Actas Dermosifiliogr. 2014;105:887–90.

34. Gaspari R, Blehar D, Mendoza M, Montoya A, Moon C, Polan D. Use of ultrasound elastography for skin and subcutaneous abscesses. J Ultrasound Med. 2009;28:855–60.

35. Cucoş M, Crişan M, Lenghel M, Dudea M, Croitoru R, Dudea S. Conventional ultrasonography and sonoelastography in the assessment of plaque psoriasis under topical corticosteroid treatment—work in progress. Med Ultrason. 2014;16:107–13.

36. Guazzaroni M, Ferrari D, Lamacchia F, Marisi V, Tatulli D, Marsico S, et al. Shear wave elastography and microvascular ultrasound in response evaluation to calcipotriol+betamethasone foam in plaque psoriasis. Postgrad Med J. 2021;97:16–22. https://doi.org/10.1136/postgradmedj-2020-138150.

37. Asil K, Yaldiz M. Diagnostic role of ultrasound elastography for nail bed involvement in psoriasis. Medicine (Baltimore). 2019;98(50):e17917. https://doi.org/10.1097/MD.0000000000017917.

38. Iznardo H, Vilarrasa E, Roé E, Puig L. Shear wave elastography as a potential tool for quantitative assessment of sinus tracts fibrosis in hidradenitis suppurativa. J Eur Acad Dermatol Venereol. 2022; https://doi.org/10.1111/jdv.18116. Epub ahead of print.

39. Iagnocco A, Kaloudi O, Perella C, Bandinelli F, Riccieri V, Vasile M, et al. Ultrasound elastography assessment of skin involvement in systemic sclerosis: Lights and shadows. J Rheumatol. 2010;37:1688–91.

40. Di Geso L, Filippucci E, Girolimetti R, Tardella M, Gutierrez M, de Angelis R, et al. Reliability of ultrasound measurements of dermal thickness at digits in systemic sclerosis: role of elastosonography. Clin Exp Rheumatol. 2011;29:926–32.

41. Tumsatan P, Uscharapong M, Srinakarin J, Nanagara R, Khunkitti W. Role of shear wave elastography ultrasound in patients with systemic sclerosis. J Ultrasound. 2022; https://doi.org/10.1007/s40477-021-00637-0. Epub ahead of print.

42. Kaya İslamoğlu ZG, Uysal E. A preliminary study on ultrasound techniques applied to cicatricial alopecia. Skin Res Technol. 2019;25:810–4. https://doi.org/10.1111/srt.12725. Epub 2019 May 29

Soft Parts: Malignant Pathology

3

Mesut Ozturk, Ahmet Peker, Enes Gurun,
and Ahmet Veysel Polat

3.1 Introduction

Radiological differentiation of malignant and benign soft tissue tumors is crucial for clinical management and optimal surgical technique. Most soft tissue tumors are benign and are resected with a preliminary diagnosis of malignancy. Before surgical resection, imaging of the tumors with radiological methods is performed, and a preliminary diagnosis is aimed to be reached whether it is malignant or benign [1, 2]. Radiography, ultrasonography (US), computed tomography (CT), magnetic resonance imaging (MRI), and positron emission tomography (PET) are imaging modalities used for diagnosis [3–7]. Among these methods, the US has advantages such as being cheap and readily available in most institutions, having high resolution and no radiation, lack of contraindication and allowing to obtain clinical history during the examination thanks to one-to-one contact with the patient [8].

Elastography is a US-based radiological imaging method. During US examination, elastic properties of the tissues can be evaluated simultaneously with US elastography. US and US elastography have been proven to be effective in the diagnosis of various organ/system diseases [9–16]. In the current literature, there are many studies investigating the diagnostic value of US and elastography in the differentiation of malignant and benign soft tissue tumors [17–26]. In this chapter, US and elastography features of malignant soft tissue tumors, the diagnostic value of US and elastography in differentiating malignant and benign soft tissue tumors are discussed and the current literature on this subject is summarized.

3.2 US Imaging of the Soft Tissue Tumors

US is the first-choice modality in the presence of imaging indication for a soft tissue tumor [27]. According to the appropriateness criteria of The American College of Radiology, it is "usually appropriate" to evaluate a soft tissue mass that is superficial or palpable as the initial imaging study. In the case of non-diagnostic US examination, MRI is "usually appropriate" for the next imaging study [27]. US is an effective imaging modality, especially in tumors located superficially on the fascia and smaller than 5 cm in size.

M. Ozturk (✉) · E. Gurun
Department of Radiology, Samsun University Faculty of Medicine, Samsun, Turkey

A. Peker
Department of Radiology, Koc University Hospitals, Istanbul, Turkey

A. V. Polat
Department of Radiology, Ondokuz Mayis University Faculty of Medicine, Samsun, Turkey

It was reported that MRI is more effective in evaluating the large tumors located deep in the fascia [28, 29]. US is very effective in the evaluation of the internal structure of the lesion, especially in the distinction between cyst and solid.

During imaging of a soft tissue tumor, the possible highest frequency probe that allows full visualization of the tumor should be chosen. Hockey stick-shaped US probes may be useful, especially for the lesions located in the face, fingers, and nails. For large lesions and deep localizations, a convex probe with low frequency may be used. When examining a soft tissue tumor with US, the anatomic location of the tumor, the location of the lesion relative to the fascia (superficial or deep), its 3-dimensions, its internal structure (echo feature, cystic or solid content, whether it contains areas of necrosis, presence of calcification), presence and the type of vascularity, the morphology of the tumor (shape, margins), and the appearance of the surrounding soft tissues should be reported [2, 30–32].

Soft tissue tumors can be located in the skin and subcutaneous tissue superficial to the superficial fascia or deep into the superficial fascia. Deep localization to the fascia was reported to be associated with malignancy [21, 23, 26, 33, 34].

Studies in the literature have reported that malignancy is more common in soft tissue tumors larger than 5 cm in diameter [18, 19, 21, 29, 35].

However, malignant soft tissue tumors can also be located superficial to the fascia and may be less than 5 cm in diameter at presentation. A solid mass with a history of rapid growth should always raise the suspicion of malignancy [36].

Color Doppler US imaging provides information about the internal vascularization of the examined tumor without contrast material administration. Giovagnoria et al. [37] investigated the color Doppler US features of soft tissue tumors and reported a classification system. According to this classification, avascular lesions were classified as type 1; lesions with blood supply from a single pole were classified as type 2; lesions with multiple peripheral blood vessels were classified as type 3; lesions with internal vascularity were classified as type 4. The sensitivity and specificity of this classification in the diagnosis of malig-

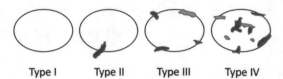

Type I   Type II   Type III   Type IV

Fig. 3.1 Giovagnoria color Doppler US classification system. Avascular lesions are classified as type I, lesions with blood supply from a single pole are classified as type II, lesions with multiple peripheral blood vessels are classified as type III, lesions with internal vascularization are classified as type IV

nant lesions were 70–90% and 75–100%, respectively [21, 37] (Fig. 3.1).

Other US features that favor malignancy include obtuse contact angle with the fascia, taller-than-wider shape, lobulated shape, indistinct or infiltrative borders, heterogeneous echo texture with intralesional cystic, necrotic and hemorrhagic components, presence of perilesional edema [38].

3.3 Elastography Acquisition Techniques of the Soft Tissue Tumors

Palpation has been one of the main examination methods in medicine for many years and is still a very important part of physical examination today. However, palpation is a subjective assessment and has limitations. Elastography attempts to overcome this limitation of palpation by evaluating the mechanical properties of tissue noninvasively. US elastography can be divided into two according to the source of force applied to the tissue: strain elastography (SE) and shear wave elastography (SWE) [39].

3.3.1 Strain Elastography

In SE, a compression force is applied to the tissue by the operator, and this compression force produces displacement or strain in the tissue [9, 40]. The harder the tissue, the lesser the strain; the softer the tissue, the greater the strain. Repetitive compression force is applied to the tissue with the US probe, and displacements in the tissue are coded with a colored elastogram map superimposed on the B-mode image [41]. In this elastogram map, tissues with higher strain are coded in red (soft), tissues with lower strain are coded in blue (hard), and tissues with moderate strain are coded in green. Malignant tumors are usually harder than benign tumors and therefore they contain more blue-colored areas [24]. The elastography color map is classified into four categories according to the amount of red, green, and blue areas and the SE visual pattern of the lesion is determined [17, 22, 42]. In this classification system, score 1 is assigned to the tumors that are predominantly green to red with small areas of blue; score 2 is assigned to the tumors that are more green than blue in the ROI; score 3 is assigned to the tumors that are more blue than green in the ROI; score 4 is assigned to the tumors that are predominantly blue with few small areas of green in the ROI (Fig. 3.2). The sensitivity, specificity, positive predictive value, and negative predictive value of this classification system in the diagnosis of malignant tumors were reported as 100%, 51.6%, 51.6%, and 100%, respectively [24]. Some authors used a 5-point visual scoring system which was suggested by Itoh et al. [17, 20, 43, 44]. In this classification system, score 1 corresponded to green color in the entire tumor, score 2 corresponded to a mosaic pattern of green and blue of the tumor, score 3 corresponded to blue in the central part and green in the peripheral part of the tumor, score 4 corresponded to blue in the entire tumor, and score 5 corresponded to blue in the entire tumor and its surrounding area (Fig. 3.3). According to these criteria scores 1–3 were categorized as benign and scores 4 and 5

were categorized as malignant. The sensitivity and specificity of this classification system in the diagnosis of malignant tumors were reported as 56% and 57%, respectively [44].

Sometimes a color map cannot be obtained from some areas of the tumor, and this situation is called "black sign." Black sign may be associated with artifacts or malignancy [45, 46]. Malignant tumors may be surrounded by a stiff tissue, causing a desmoplastic reaction around them due to infiltration. This desmoplastic reaction is also coded blue in the elastogram map and is called the "blue halo sign" [43, 47].

SE elastogram map may be affected by the force applied too heavily or too gently, due to the nonlinearity of the tissue elasticity graph. Therefore, SE is operator dependent. In addition, most systems in SE do not give objective numerical values and evaluate the elasticity of the examined tissue by comparing it with the elasticity of an adjacent tissue [9, 40, 41]. Moreover, the lesion may not be compressed because of a hard tissue adjacent to it and strain may not be created in the examined tissue, which is called the "egg shell effect" [30, 48].

In SE, the ratio of adjacent fat tissue strain to the lesion strain results in strain ratio (SR). In the studies by Hahn et al. [17], Riishede et al. [20], and Li et al. [24], the SR of malignant and benign soft tissue tumors significantly differed. The sensitivity and specificity of the SR in the differentiation were reported as 93.8%, 80.5%, 65.2%, and 97.1%, respectively, for a cut-off SR value of 2.29 [24]. Cohen et al. [44] and Dou et al. [22] reported no significant difference between the SR of benign and malignant soft tissue tumors.

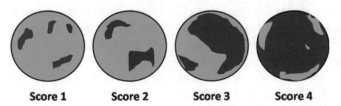

Score 1   **Score 2**   **Score 3**   **Score 4**

Fig. 3.2 Illustration of the 4-point strain elastography color map scoring system. Score 1 is assigned to the tumors predominantly green to red with small areas of blue; score 2 is assigned to the tumors more green than blue in the ROI; score 3 is assigned to the tumors more blue than green in the ROI; score 4 is assigned to the tumors predominantly blue with few small areas of green

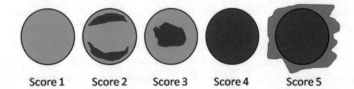

Score 1   Score 2   Score 3   Score 4   Score 5

Fig. 3.3 Illustration of the 5-point strain elastography color map scoring system. Score 1 corresponds to green color in the entire tumor, score 2 corresponds to a mosaic pattern of green and blue of the tumor, score 3 corre- sponds to blue in the central part and green in the periph- eral part of the tumor, score 4 corresponds to blue in the entire tumor, and score 5 corresponds to blue in the entire tumor and its surrounding area

3.3.2 Shear Wave Elastography

In SWE, the mechanical compression force applied to the tissue is provided by the acoustic radiation force produced by the US probe [9, 21]. Therefore, shear wave elastography has been reported to be more objective and repro- ducible. The absolute elasticity of the tissue can be determined with SWE. The quantitative elas- ticity measurement value is expressed as shear wave velocity (SWV) in meters per second (m/s) or shear modulus calculation in kilopascals (kPa).

Studies in the literature reported variable results for the efficacy of SWV measurements in differentiating benign and malignant tumors. In studies by Li et al. [33] and Ohshika et al. [23], SWV measurements were able to differentiate benign and malignant soft tissue tumors, whereas in other studies SWV measurements were not significantly different between benign and malig- nant lesions [18, 19, 21, 26, 34].

The solid and hypervascular area of the tumor should be examined while SWE examination [8]. With SWE, an elastogram map is also obtained as in SE, and red color encodes hard areas and blue color encodes soft areas. Since most soft tissue sarcomas have very variable histopathological features such as necrosis, hemorrhage, and calci- fication, blue and red colors are often displayed together in the same lesion. The sensitivity, spec- ificity, positive predictive value, and negative predictive value of the visual scoring system of SWE were reported as 61.9%, 90%, 68.4%, and 87.1%, respectively [33].

3.4 Clinical Applications of US and US Elastography for Evaluation of Malignant Soft Tissue Tumors and Literature Review

Soft tissue tumors consist of various cell types originating from the mesenchyme or neuroecto- derm. Therefore, it has a wide variety of subtypes according to the tissue of origin [49]. The most common malignant soft tissue tumors in adult patients are pleomorphic sarcoma and liposar- coma [8, 50]. The most common malignant soft tissue sarcoma in children is rhabdomyosarcoma [51].

There are many studies evaluating the diag- nostic value of US elastography in the diagnosis of soft tissue tumors [17–24, 26, 33, 34, 42, 44]. Variable results have been reported in these stud- ies (Table 3.1).

Park et al. [42] evaluated 103 soft tissue tumors with US and SE. They had 28 malignant tumors. SE evaluation was based on a visual analysis from score 1 (very soft, high elasticity) to score 4 (very hard, low elasticity). Tumor size, margin irregularity, shape, and echogenicity were assessed as the US features. The authors reported that malignant tumors exhibited higher SE scores than benign tumors ($p = 0.001$). While 82% of malignant tumors had a score of 3 or 4, 46% of benign tumors had SE scores of 3 or 4. In their study, malignant tumors were significantly larger in size than benign tumors ($p = 0.005$). Echotexture of the lesion was significantly asso- ciated with the malignant diagnosis, as malignant

Table 3.1 Characteristics of studies in the literature investigating the value of US and US elastography in the diagnosis of malignant and benign soft tissue tumors

The study	Number of malignant STTs/Total number of STTs (%)	Histopathologic diagnosis of the malignant STTs	Elastography technique used	Elastography comments	US evaluation	US evaluation comments
Park et al. [42]	28/103 (27.2%)	• Lymphoma (n = 5). • Metastatic lymph node (n = 4). • Malignant melanoma (n = 4). • Soft tissue metastasis (n = 3). • Myxofibrosarcoma (n = 3). • Kaposi sarcoma (n = 2). • Undifferentiated pleomorphic sarcoma (n = 2). • Malignant peripheral nerve sheet tumor (n = 1). • Merkel cell carcinoma (n = 1). • Synovial sarcoma (n = 1). • Squamous cell carcinoma (n = 1). • Basal cell carcinoma (n = 1).	• SE; VGS.	• Scores 3 and 4 were observed in 82% of malignant tumors and 46% of benign tumors; $p = 0.001$.	• Lesion size. • Margin irregularity. • Shape. • Echogenicity.	• Malignant lesions were significantly larger than benign lesions ($p = 0.005$). • Hypo—Mixed echogenicity was significantly associated with malignancy (100% of malignant tumors vs. 68% of benign tumors, $p = 0.006$). • Margins and shape was not associated with malignancy ($p = 0.092$ and 0.887).

(continued)

Table 3.1 (continued)

The study	Number of malignant STTs/Total number of STTs (%)	Histopathologic diagnosis of the malignant STTs	Elastography technique used	Elastography comments	US evaluation	US evaluation comments
Li et al. [33]	21/81 (25.9%)	• Metastasis ($n = 2$). • Myxoid liposarcoma ($n = 3$). • Plexiform fibrohistiocytic tumor ($n = 1$). • Myxofibrosarcoma ($n = 1$). • Synovial sarcoma ($n = 2$). • Rhabdomyosarcoma ($n = 1$). • Fusocellular sarcoma ($n = 4$). • Lymphoma ($n = 2$). • Solitary fibrous tumor ($n = 1$). • Malignant mesenchymoma ($n = 2$). • Undifferentiated sarcoma ($n = 2$).	• SWE; E_{max}, E_{mean}, E_{min}, E_{sd}. • SWE; VGS.	SWE measurements, benign vs. malignant: • E_{max}: 3.8 vs. 5.76; $p < 0.001$. • E_{mean}: 2.40 vs. 3.20; $p < 0.001$. • E_{min}: 1.40 vs. 0.50; $p < 0.001$. • E_{sd}: 0.42 vs. 0.88; $p < 0.001$. SWE VGS, benign vs. malignant: • Patterns 3 and 4 were observed in 61.9% of malignant tumors and 10% of benign tumors, $p < 0.001$.	• Depth. • Margin. • Echogenicity. • Vascularity.	• Depth was significantly associated with malignancy (66.7% of malignant tumors vs. 38.3% of benign tumors, $p = 0.041$). • Infiltrative margin was significantly associated with malignancy (42.9% malignant tumors vs. 10% benign tumors, $p = 0.002$). • Hypoechoic appearance was significantly associated with malignancy (100% of malignant tumors vs. 63.3% of benign tumors, $p = 0.002$). • Disorganized power Doppler signal was associated with malignancy (61.9% of malignant tumors vs. 41.7% benign tumors, $p = 0.024$).
Pass et al. [18]	39/105 (37.1%)	NA	• SWE; SWV in transverse and longitudinal planes.	• There was no statistically significant difference between SWV of benign and malignant lesions.	• Echogenicity. • Mass texture. • Vascularity. • Depth. • B-mode subjective classification.	• Hypo or mixed echogenicity was significantly associated with malignancy (97.7% of malignant tumors vs. 86.9% of benign tumors, $p = 0.025$). • Disorganized vascularity was significantly associated with malignancy (56.8% of malignant tumors vs. 19.7% of benign tumors, $p = 0.004$). • Mass texture and depth were not associated with malignancy ($p = 0.777$ and $p = 0.883$). • B-mode subjective classification had 76.9% sensitivity and 78.8% specificity.

Pass et al. [19]	15/50 (30%)	• Sarcoma ($n = 10$). • Metastases ($n = 5$).	• SWE; longitudinal SWV, transverse SWV.	• Longitudinal and transverse SWV measurements were not significantly different between benign and malignant tumors ($p = 0.095$ and $p = 0.413$).	• Consensus US reading.	• Consensus US reading had 73.3% sensitivity and 77.1% specificity.
Hahn et al. [17]	33/73 (45.2%)	• Metastases ($n = 18$). • Lymphoma ($n = 4$). • Malignant melanoma ($n = 4$). • Malignant nerve tumor ($n = 1$). • Plasmocytoma ($n = 1$). • Chondrosarcoma ($n = 1$). • Myxoid liposarcoma ($n = 1$). • Angiosarcoma ($n = 1$). • Ewing sarcoma ($n = 1$). • Extraskeletal osteosarcoma ($n = 1$).	• SE, 5-point visual scale elasticity score. • SE, strain ratio.	• Elasticity scores and strain ratios were significantly different between benign and malignant tumors ($p = 0.048$ and $p = 0.003$).	NA	
Riishede et al. [20]	19/61 (31.1%)	• Liposarcoma ($n = 4$). • Undifferentiated sarcoma ($n = 2$). • Grade III sarcoma ($n = 1$). • Chondrosarcoma ($n = 1$). • Osteosarcoma ($n = 1$). • Myxofibrosarcoma ($n = 1$). • Metastasis ($n = 5$). • Lymphoma ($n = 4$).	• SE, strain ratio. • SE, visual score. • SE, strain histograms.	• Mean strain ratio of malignant (1.94) and benign (1.35) lesions were significantly different ($p = 0.043$). • Mean visual scores of malignant and benign lesions were not significantly different ($p = 0.414$). • Mean strain histograms of malignant and benign lesions were not significantly different ($p = 0.317$).	NA	

(continued)

Table 3.1 (continued)

The study	Number of malignant STTs/Total number of STTs (%)	Histopathologic diagnosis of the malignant STTs	Elastography technique used	Elastography comments	US evaluation	US evaluation comments
Li et al. [24]	17/61 (27.9%)	• Metastatic carcinoma ($n = 10$). • Lymphoma ($n = 3$). • Malignant melanoma ($n = 2$). • Liposarcoma ($n = 1$). • Myeloma ($n = 1$).	• SE, strain ratio. • SE, visual score.	• Mean strain ratio of benign (1.8) and malignant (5.42) tumors were significantly different ($p < 0.001$). • Mean elasticity score of benign (2.03) and malignant (3.13) were significantly different ($p < 0.001$).	NA	
Cohen et al. [44]	56/137 (40.9%)	• Sarcoma ($n = 30$). • Metastasis ($n = 12$). • Lymphoma ($n = 11$). • Gastrointestinal stromal tumor ($n = 1$). • Multiple myelomatosis ($n = 1$). • Malignant solitary fibrous tumor ($n = 1$).	• SE, strain ratio. • SE, visual score.	• Mean strain ratio of benign (2.30) and malignant (2.66) tumors were not significantly different ($p = 0.30$). • Mean elasticity score of benign (3.16) and malignant (3.49) were significantly different ($p = 0.043$).	• Lesion size.	• Malignant lesions were significantly larger in size than benign lesions (6.55 cm vs. 5.5 cm, $p = 0.007$).

| Winn et al. [26] | 61/148 (41.2%) | • Myxofibrosarcoma (*n* = 12).
 • Pleomorphic sarcoma (*n* = 8).
 • Liposarcoma (*n* = 9).
 • Leiomyosarcoma (*n* = 3).
 • Synovial sarcoma (*n* = 3).
 • Spindle cell sarcoma (*n* = 3).
 • Malignant nerve tumor (*n* = 1).
 • Undifferentiated sarcoma (*n* = 1).
 • Ewing's sarcoma (*n* = 1).
 • Chondrosarcoma (*n* = 1).
 • Metastasis (*n* = 7).
 • Lymphoma (*n* = 7).
 • Malignant melanoma (*n* = 3).
 • Merkel cell carcinoma (*n* = 3). | • SWE, SWV. | • Malignant tumors trended to have slower SWV (3.73 m/s) compared to benign tumors (4.36), however, the difference was not statistically different (*p* = 0.06). | • Lesion size.
 • Depth.
 • Echogenicity.
 • Margins.
 • Vascularity.
 • Posterior acoustic enhancement. | • Malignant lesions were significantly larger in size than benign lesions (79.3 ml vs. 19.6 mL; *p* = 0.001).
 • Depth of the lesion was not significantly different between benign and malignant lesions (7.7 mm vs. 6.3 mm; *p* = 0.2).
 • Margin was not significantly different between benign and malignant lesions.
 • Malignant lesions demonstrated greater vascularity than benign lesions (*p* < 0.001).
 • Presence of posterior acoustic enhancement was not significantly different between benign and malignant lesions. |

(continued)

Table 3.1 (continued)

The study	Number of malignant STTs/Total number of STTs (%)	Histopathologic diagnosis of the malignant STTs	Elastography technique used	Elastography comments	US evaluation	US evaluation comments
Tavare et al. [34]	79/206 (38%)	• Liposarcoma (n = 22). • Spindle cell sarcoma (n = 11). • Metastasis (n = 9). • Lymphoma (n = 7). • Malignant nerve tumor (n = 4). • Leiomyosarcoma (n = 5). • Dermatofibrosarcoma protuberans (n = 2). • Myxofibrosarcoma (n = 2). • Alveolar soft tissue sarcoma (n = 1). • Ewing sarcoma (n = 1). • Fibrosarcoma (n = 1). • Myxoinflammatory fibroblastic sarcoma (n = 1). • Synovial sarcoma (n = 2). • Invasive ductal carcinoma (n = 1). • Plasmacytoma (n = 1). • Merkel cell tumor (n = 3). • Solitary fibrous tumor (n = 3). • Aggressive fibromatosis (n = 1).	• SWE, SWV.	• Mean SWV of malignant and benign lesions were not significantly different (2.23 vs. 2.31, $p = 0.54$). • SWV showed good diagnostic accuracy for lesions classified as benign or probably benign by US alone. • SWV did not provide substantive diagnostic information for lesions classified as probably malignant of malignant.	• B-mode visual assessment. • Lesion size. • Heterogeneity. • Necrosis present. • Echotexture. • Doppler. • Position.	• The sensitivity and specificity of B-mode visual assessment were 80.6% and 80.3%, respectively. • Malignant lesions (94.7 mL) were significantly larger than benign lesions (30.1 mL, $p < 0.001$). • Necrosis was significantly more common in malignant lesions (41% vs. 17%, $p < 0.001$). • Hypoechoic appearance was significantly more common in malignant lesions (61% vs. 43%, $p = 0.02$). • Disorganized Doppler sign was significantly more common in malignant lesions (71% vs. 24%, $p < 0.001$). • Mixed position was significantly more common in malignant lesions (14% vs. %1, $p = 0.002$).

| Ohshika et al. [23] | 47/167 (28.1%) | • Myxofibrosarcoma (*n* = 14).
• Liposarcoma (*n* = 7).
• Undifferentiated pleomorphic sarcoma (*n* = 4).
• Soft tissue metastasis (*n* = 4).
• Rhabdomyosarcoma (*n* = 3).
• Leiomyosarcoma (*n* = 3).
• Extraskeletal myxoid chondrosarcoma (*n* = 2).
• Extraskeletal osteosarcoma (*n* = 2).
• Synovial sarcoma (*n* = 2).
• High grade sarcoma (*n* = 2).
• Malignant lymphoma (*n* = 2).
• Low-grade fibromyxoid sarcoma (*n* = 1).
• Clear cell sarcoma (*n* = 1). | • SWE, maximal SWV. | • Median maximal SWV of malignant lesions (8.3) was significantly different than the that of the intermediate (7) and benign (6.1) lesions ($p < 0.05$). | • Lesion size.
• Depth. | • Median tumor size in the intermediate (7.8 cm) and malignant (8.0) group was significantly larger than that of the benign (5) group ($p < 0.001$); however, there was no significant difference between the intermediate and malignant group ($p = 0.109$).
• Ratio of deep lesion was significantly higher in the intermediate and malignant groups ($p = 0.005$). |

(continued)

Table 3.1 (continued)

The study	Number of malignant STTs/Total number of STTs (%)	Histopathologic diagnosis of the malignant STTs	Elastography technique used	Elastography comments	US evaluation	US evaluation comments
Dou et al. [22]	36/83 (43.4%)	• Metastasis (*n* = 5). • Liposarcoma (*n* = 4). • Leiomyosarcoma (*n* = 3). • Lymphoma (*n* = 3). • Synoviosarcoma (*n* = 3). • Melanoma (*n* = 2). • Liposarcoma (*n* = 5). • Malignant schwannoma (*n* = 2). • Rhabdosarcoma (*n* = 2). • Malignant giant cell tumor (*n* = 1). • Pleomorphic sarcoma (*n* = 1). • Squamous carcinoma (*n* = 1). • Aggressive fibromatosis (*n* = 1).	• SE, strain ratio. • SE, elasticity score.	• Mean strain ratio malignant and benign tumors did not differ significantly (2.33 vs. 1.99, *p* = 0.517). • Mean elastography scores of malignant and benign lesions were significantly different (2.81 vs. 2.36, *p* = 0.011).	• Maximum diameter. • Echogenicity. • Tail sign. • Cystic component. • Doppler score. • Depth. • Heterogeneity. • Margin. • Elastography size to B-mode size.	• Superficial localization was significantly more common in benign tumors (34% vs. 5.6%, *p* = 0.003). • Heterogeneous appearance was significantly more common in malignant tumors than in benign tumors (94.4% vs. 74.5%, *p* = 0.016). • Irregular margin was significantly more common in malignant tumors than in benign tumors (76.9% vs. 19.1%, *p* < 0.001). • Elastography size to B-mode size >1 was significantly more common in malignant tumors than in benign tumors (86.1% vs. 29.8%, *p* < 0.001).

| Ozturk et al. [21] | 37/109 (33.9%) | • Metastasis ($n = 7$).
• Myxofibrosarcoma ($n = 6$).
• Synovial sarcoma ($n = 3$).
• Angiosarcoma ($n = 2$).
• Leiomyosarcoma ($n = 2$).
• Lymphoma ($n = 2$).
• Malignant nerve tumor ($n = 2$).
• Rhabdomyosarcoma ($n = 2$).
• Undifferentiated spindle cell sarcoma ($n = 2$).
• Undifferentiated sarcoma ($n = 2$).
• Undifferentiated pleomorphic sarcoma ($n = 2$).
• Liposarcoma ($n = 2$).
• Epithelioid sarcoma ($n = 1$).
• Fibrosarcoma ($n = 1$).
• Undifferentiated epithelioid sarcoma ($n = 1$). | • SWE, SWV_{mean}.
• SWE, SWV_{max}. | • Median SWV_{mean} of malignant (2.87) and benign (2.68) lesions did not differ significantly ($p = 0.271$).
• Median SWV_{max} of malignant (3.30) and benign (3.05) lesions did not differ significantly ($p = 0.402$). | • Consensus US reading.
• Lesion size.
• Localization.
• Echogenicity.
• Texture.
• Cystic component.
• Margin.
• Doppler findings. | • The sensitivity and specificity of consensus US readings were 91.9% and 72.2%.
• Lesion size significantly differed between benign and malignant lesions (maximum diameter 7.5 cm vs. 4.1 cm, $p < 0.001$).
• Deep localization was significantly more common in malignant lesions (86.5% vs. 52.8%, $p = 0.001$).
• Hypoechoic appearance was significantly more common in malignant lesions (89.2% vs. 62.5%, $p = 0.003$).
• Cystic component was significantly more common in malignant lesions (54.1% vs. 29.2%, $p = 0.011$).
• Ill-defined margins were significantly more common in malignant lesions (89.2% vs. 58.3%, $p = 0.001$).
• Type 3 and 4 Doppler patterns were more common in malignant lesions (70.3% vs. 25%, $p < 0.001$). |

STTs soft tissue tumors, *SE* strain elastography, *SWE* shear wave elastography, *SWV* shear wave velocity, *VGS* visual grading system

tumors significantly demonstrated a higher incidence of mixed echogenicity.

Li et al. [33] evaluated 81 histopathologically proven soft tissue tumors using US and SWE. Their study included 21 malignant cases (25.9%). In the authors' study, larger lesion size and deep localization were significantly associated with malignant pathology. US features of infiltrative margins, hypoechogenicity, and disorganized power Doppler signal were significantly associated with malignant pathology. In the multivariate analysis, infiltrative margins and size were the strongest predictors of malignancy with Odds ratios of 4.470 and 1.046. SWE measurements of E_{max}, E_{mean}, E_{min}, and E_{sd} were significantly different between benign and malignant lesions. E_{sd} was the strongest predictor of malignancy with an Odds ratio of 9.047.

Pass et al. [18] evaluated the grayscale characteristics of the 105 soft tissue tumors and investigated whether the SWE technique contributed to the differentiation of benign and malignant lesions. In their study, lesion echogenicity and power Doppler features were significantly different between benign and malignant lesions. Mass texture and depth were not associated with malignancy. Larger lesion size and advanced patient age were also found to be associated with malignancy, but the SWE technique did not contribute to histological differentiation. Although the SWV values of malignant lesions (2.57 m/s) were found to be lower than the SWV values of benign lesions (2.94 m/s), this difference was not statistically significant. Consensus US reading of the lesions demonstrated 76.9% sensitivity and 78.8% specificity. The authors also performed a complex statistical analysis by adding SWV measurements to the US classification to assess if SWE improves diagnostic accuracy. However, adding SWE measurements to the consensus US reading did not improve the diagnostic accuracy.

In another study, Pass et al. [19] examined 50 soft tissue masses with the VTQ function of SWE. In their study, longitudinal and transverse SWV measurements of malignant lesions were not significantly different that those of the benign lesions ($p = 0.095$ and $p = 0.413$). The authors also evaluated the US features of the lesions,

such as echogenicity, texture, lesion size, vascularity, and lesion localization. According to the US features, malignant lesions tended to be larger (4 times larger than benign lesions), hyperechoic (26.7% of malignant lesions vs. 5.7% of benign lesions), and homogenous in appearance (46.7% of malignant lesions vs. 22.9% of benign lesions). In their study, consensus US reading of the lesions by two radiologists demonstrated 73.3% sensitivity and 77.1% specificity.

Hahn et al. [17] investigated the value of SE in the differentiation of benign and malignant soft tissue masses in a series of 73 patients. There were 40 benign and 33 malignant cases. In this study, the strain ratio of malignant lesions (0.49 ± 0.45) was found to be statistically significantly smaller than that of benign lesions (1.03 ± 0.93, p = 0.003). They also evaluated the visual elasticity score and reported that the elasticity scores were significantly different between benign and malignant tumors (p = 0.048). The mean elasticity scores of benign tumors were 3.08 ± 1.44 and the mean elasticity score of malignant tumors were 3.76 ± 0.97. The authors compared the diagnostic accuracy of elasticity score and strain ratio and reported no significant difference between these two measurements ($p = 0.304$).

Riishede et al. [20] examined 61 soft tissue tumors with SE. Their series included 19 malignant tumors. In their study, the mean SR of benign and malignant lesions significantly differed (1.35 vs. 1.94, $p = 0.043$). In terms of visual scoring and strain histogram, there was no significant difference between benign and malignant tumors ($p = 0.414$ and $p = 0.317$). The authors excluded the benign (lipoma) and malignant (liposarcoma) fat-containing tumors from the study cohort and performed the statistical analysis again. For the second analysis, the mean SR of benign and malignant lesions were again significantly different with a lower p value (1.33 vs. 2.13, $p = 0.014$). Visual scoring and strain histogram were again not significantly different between benign and malignant tumors ($p = 0.352$ and $p = 0.359$).

Li et al. [24] evaluated 61 patients with superficial masses and found significantly increased

SR values (5.42 vs 1.8) and elasticity scores (3.13 vs. 2.03) in malignant tumors ($p < 0.001$). Their study was composed of 44 benign and 17 malignant tumors. With a SR of >2.3 as the optimal threshold value, the sensitivity and specificity of SR for diagnosing a malignant tumor were 93.8% and 80.5%, respectively. On the other hand, an elasticity score of ≥ 3 as the optimal threshold value, the sensitivity and specificity of the elasticity score for diagnosing a malignant mass were 100% and 52%, respectively. Furthermore, the diagnostic performances of these two techniques were not significantly different ($p > 0.05$).

Cohen et al. [44] evaluated 137 lesions (81 benign, 56 malignant) with strain elastography. In their study, they obtained statistically significant results between benign and malignant lesions with Tsukuba Elasticity Score (TES) scoring system (3.16 and 3.49, respectively; $p = 0.043$). The mean strain ratio of benign and malignant lesions was not significantly different (2.30 vs. 2.66, $p = 0.30$). The authors' study included 32 fat-containing benign tumors and 5 fat-containing malignant tumors. They excluded these cases from the study cohort and performed the statistical analysis again. In the second analysis, the mean TES score and mean strain ratio of benign and malignant lesions were not significantly different (3.56 vs. 3.54, $p = 0.92$; 2.68 vs. 2.75, $p = 0.88$). The authors reported that the mean size of malignant lesions was significantly larger than that of the benign lesions (6.55 cm vs. 5.5 cm, $p = 0.007$).

Winn et al. [26] evaluated 148 soft tissue tumors with SWE. There were 61 malignant tumors. In their study, malignant lesions trended toward a slower SWV (3.73 m/s, ln 1.25 m/s) compared to benign lesions (4.36 m/s, ln 1.37 m/s); however, this did not meet statistical significance owing to the overlap between the groups ($p = 0.06$). The authors compared the lesion size, depth of the lesion, echogenicity, margins, vascularity, and posterior acoustic enhancement between benign and malignant soft tissue tumors. The authors reported that malignant lesions were significantly greater in size and demonstrated greater vascularity. Lesion depth, margin characteristics, echogenicity, and poste-rior acoustic enhancement were not significantly different between benign and malignant soft tissue tumors.

Tavare et al. [34] evaluated 206 lesions of which 79 were malignant. The mean SWV of the malignant lesions (2.23 m/s) was not significantly different than that of the benign lesions (2.31 m/s, $p = 0.54$). Their results showed that while SWV alone was not diagnostic for malignancy, it improved the diagnostic accuracy of imaging-based US classification when the lesions were initially believed to be benign or probably benign. No additional benefit of SWE was seen when assessment based on US alone was indicative of a possible or definite malignancy. In their study, larger lesion size, presence of necrosis, hypoechoic appearance, and disorganized Doppler signal were significantly associated with malignancy.

Ohshika et al. [23] found significant a difference between malignant, intermediate, and benign soft tissue tumors. The authors evaluated 47 malignant, 21 intermediate, and 99 benign tumors. The mean maximal SWV of malignant lesions (8.3 m/s, range: 7.9–8.7) was significantly different than that of the benign (6.1 m/s, range: 3.4–7.7) and intermediate (7.0 m/s, range: 5.9–7.6) lesions ($p < 0.05$). The authors reported that the tumor size in the intermediate and malignant groups was significantly larger than that of the benign group ($p < 0.001$), however, there was no significant difference between the intermediate and malignant groups ($p = 0.109$). Intermediate and malignant lesions were more likely to localize deep into the fascia ($p = 0.005$).

Dou et al. [22] evaluated 36 malignant and 47 nonmalignant tumors with SE. The authors found no significant difference between the malignant and nonmalignant groups in terms of mean SR (2.33 ± 2.33 and 1.99 ± 2.37, $p = 0.517$). In their study, they found a significant difference between the mean elasticity scores of malignant and benign lesions (2.81 ± 0.71 and 2.36 ± 0.82, $p = 0.011$). The authors also evaluated the US features of the lesions. Localization to the fascia ($p = 0.003$), heterogeneity ($p = 0.016$), and tumor margin ($p < 0.001$) were significantly different between benign and malignant tumors whereas echogenicity (p = 0.258), cystic component (p = 0.145), Doppler scores (p = 0.054), and Tail sign (p = 0.128) did not differ. Elastography size to B-mode size was significantly different between benign and malignant tumors (p < 0.001).

Ozturk et al. [21] assessed the mean and maximum SWV of 37 malignant and 72 benign soft tissue tumors with SWE. Median SWV_{mean} and median SWV_{max} of the malignant lesions (2.87 and 3.30) were not significantly different than those of the benign lesions (2.68 and 3.05; p = 0.271 and p = 0.402, respectively). In their study, larger lesion size, deep localization, hypoechoic appearance, ill-defined margins, and type 3 and 4 Doppler patterns were significantly more common in malignant tumors.

3.5 WHO Classification of Malignant Soft Tissue Tumors

3.5.1 Malignant Adipocytic Tumors

Malignant adipocytic tumors group contains liposarcoma. Liposarcoma is the second most common malignant soft tissue tumor. Patients are often between the ages of 40 and 60 years. There are well-differentiated, myxoid, pleomorphic, dedifferentiated, and myxoid pleomorphic subtypes [49]. The most commonly seen is the well-differentiated liposarcoma which makes up approximately half of these tumors [52]. Up to 75% of these tumors are localized in the deep soft tissues of the extremities, especially in the thigh region. Moreover, it is most commonly seen in the retroperitoneum, upper extremity, trunk, and head and neck, respectively. Clinically, they appear as painless, slow-growing masses. The tumor may appear as a lipoma on radiological imaging, but care should be taken to the presence of thick (>2 mm) or irregular septa. The enhancement of these septa is slightly more pronounced than the thin septa of a lipoma. Myxoid liposarcoma is the second most common type of liposarcoma. This subtype includes both myxoid tissue and round cell components. If the lesion consists predominantly of round cells, an intermediate signal will be seen on both T1 and T2-weighted images. T2 signal is high in the myxoid portions of the tumor due to the high water content. Rarely, the lesion will appear as a cyst-like mass with a homogeneous high T2 signal. Post-contrast imaging can help differentiate this lesion from a cyst by showing enhancement.

Less common subtypes of liposarcoma include pleomorphic, dedifferentiated, and mixed types. Pleomorphic liposarcomas are large, multinodular, well-demarcated tumors that contain areas of internal hemorrhage and necrosis on imaging. As these tumors contain relatively little adipose tissue, diagnosis with imaging is often difficult. Although dedifferentiated liposarcomas show similar imaging features as well-differentiated liposarcomas, they also contain soft tissue nodules larger than 1 cm that represent the dedifferentiated portion of the tumor.

Most of the malignant adipocytic tumors demonstrate macroscopic fat tissue on radiologic imaging. However, pleomorphic liposarcoma might not show evidence of macroscopic or microscopic fat on CT and MRI [53]. On CT and MRI examinations, it is recognized by the presence of fat-free septa or nodular areas in addition to areas containing adipose tissue. Adipose tissue content is inversely proportional to malignancy; as the adipose tissue content decreases, the probability of the mass being malignant increases. After IV contrast administration, contrast enhancement is seen in the septa and nodular areas.

On US examination, the appearance of liposarcomas depends on the histological type. Well-differentiated liposarcomas appear as hyperechoic well-circumscribed masses. This appearance is non-specific and similar to lipoma. Myxoid liposarcomas appear as heterogeneous hypoechoic masses with infiltrative margins. Anechoic areas can be observed in the myxoid stroma of the tumor due to mucinous components. The lesions may contain hyperechoic components depending on the presence of the amount of fat tissue. Differentiated liposarcoma is usually observed as multilobulated areas with low echogenicity. While hypervascularity is observed in the dedifferentiated region in Doppler images, there is little or no vascularity in the well-differentiated areas. Pleomorphic liposarcomas present as a heterogeneous mass consisting of many hyper and hypoechoic nodules.

Fat tissue results in lower SWV measurements. In the study by Winn et al. [26], the log-transformed mean SWV of the fatty soft tissue tumors was significantly lower than that of the non-fatty soft tissue tumors (1.01 vs. 1.34 m/s, $p = 0.01$). On the other hand, log-transformed SWV of malignant and benign fat-containing soft tissue tumors did not differ significantly (1.05 vs. 0.96 m/s, $p = 0.69$).

3.5.2 Malignant Fibroblastic and Myofibroblastic Tumors

Malignant solitary fibrous tumor, fibrosarcoma, myxofibrosarcoma, low-grade fibromyxoid sarcoma, and sclerosing epithelioid fibrosarcoma are malignant fibroblastic tumors.

Solitary fibrous tumors (SFT) are rare neoplasms of mesenchymal origin. Overall, approximately 15–20% of SFTs are malignant [54]. In US, SFTs often present as a hypoechoic mass. On CT, SFTs often appear as well-circumscribed masses that compress the adjacent tissues and organs. It is difficult to distinguish benign and malignant SFTs radiologically. It may include necrosis, bleeding, or cystic areas. On T1-weighted images, SFTs usually demonstrate an intermediate, heterogeneous signal; on T2-weighted images, they are seen as hyperintense lesions with flow voids areas. Subacute bleeding areas are seen as increased signal on T1-weighted images. On the fat-suppressed post-contrast T1-weighted image, intense heterogeneous enhancement in the arterial phase and progressive enhancement in the venous phase is observed, which are consistent with the dense fibrous content of the tumor [55, 56].

Adult fibrosarcoma is seen in 30–55 years old patients, myxofibrosarcoma is seen in elderly patients. On CT, fibrosarcomas are usually observed as poorly circumscribed isodense tumors that show mild contrast enhancement after contrast administration. These tumors show mild to moderate enhancement on MRI after gadolinium administration and have low to moderate signal intensity on all sequences [57].

Myxofibrosarcomas usually present as a painless growing soft tissue mass in the extremities. On US, they appear as nodular-multinodular hypoechoic soft tissue masses with heterogeneous internal structures. Internal septa, fascial extension (tail sing), and internal vascularization on color Doppler US can be seen. They can mimic benign lesions, and it is difficult to distinguish using US features [58] (Figs. 3.4 and 3.5).

Low-grade fibromyxoid sarcoma appears on CT as a heterogeneous mass with hypoattenuating components within the muscles. It may contain internal calcification [59].

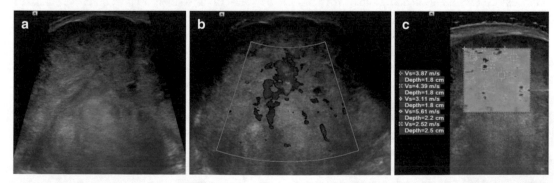

Fig. 3.4 A 61-year-old man with a soft tissue mass in his left arm. The mass is located deep in the fascia, 8 cm in its largest dimension. The mass is hypoechoic and heterogeneous in echotexture (**a**). It demonstrates type IV vascularity in Doppler examination (**b**). SWE examination and SWV measurement of the lesion is demonstrated (**c**). Histopathological examination revealed a myxofibrosarcoma

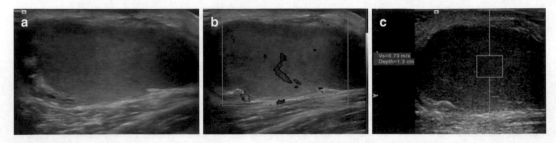

Fig. 3.5 A 39-year-old woman with a soft tissue mass in her right shoulder. The mass is located superficial to the fascia, 5 cm in its largest dimension. The mass is slightly hypoechoic in echotexture and demonstrates type III vas-cularity in Doppler examination (**a** and **b**). SWE examination and SWV measurement of the lesion is demonstrated (**c**). Histopathological examination revealed a myxofibrosarcoma

In the study by Winn et al. [26], there was no significant difference between the log-transformed mean SWV of fibrous and non-fibrous soft tissue tumors (1.39 vs. 1.29 m/s, $p = 0.34$). Furthermore, the SWV of malignant and benign fibrous tumors did not differ significantly (1.25 vs. 1.54 m/s, $p = 0.14$).

3.5.3 Malignant Vascular Tumors

This group includes epithelioid hemangioendothelioma and angiosarcoma. Epithelioid hemangioendothelioma usually occurs in adults and it is located in the deep soft tissues of the extremities. It can also be seen in other areas such as the lung, liver, and breast. On US examination, they are seen as hypoechoic or hyperechoic masses containing cystic areas. Arteriovenous shunts can be demonstrated on the Doppler examination. MRI features are similar to hemangioma. MRI often shows low-to-moderate signal intensity on T1-weighted images and high signal intensity on T2-weighted images and homogeneous contrast enhancement after gadolinium injection [60].

Angiosarcomas are malignant soft tissue tumors that can arise in deep or superficial soft tissues. Deep lesions may develop due to foreign body, radiotherapy, or chronic lymphedema. On contrast-enhanced CT, angiosarcoma typically appears as an irregularly enhancing soft tissue mass. On MRI, angiosarcomas are seen with intermediate signal intensity on T1-weighted images and high signal intensity on T2-weighted images and infiltrate into adjacent tissues. On T1-weighted images, there may be hyperintense areas representing hemorrhage [61]. Angiosarcomas associated with chronic lymphedema are called Stewart-Treves syndrome.

3.5.4 Malignant Smooth Muscle Tumors

This group includes leiomyosarcoma. It occurs in middle-aged adults and is twice as common in women as in men [62]. It can be seen in subcutaneous tissue or in the intramuscular area. Deeply localized ones are most commonly seen in the retroperitoneum. Those with superficial localization are mostly seen in the upper extremities and between the ages of 50 and 60 years. The imaging features are quite non-specific. Depending on the aggression of the lesion, it may contain cystic and necrotic areas. On US examination, they appear as well-circumscribed, hypoechoic, vascularized masses. This appearance can be confused with hemangioma. On MRI, they demonstrate an intermediate signal on T1-weighted images, a high signal on T2-weighted images, and marked enhancement after gadolinium injection. On CT, central hypodense areas that usually represent necrosis can be seen [63].

3.5.5 Malignant Skeletal Muscle Tumors

According to the WHO classification, malignant skeletal muscle tumors are grouped as embryonal rhabdomyosarcoma, alveolar rhabdomyosar-coma, pleomorphic rhabdomyosarcoma, and spindle cell/sclerosing rhabdomyosarcoma. Rhabdomyosarcoma is the most common malig-nant soft tissue tumor in childhood. It constitutes 3–5% of all childhood malignancies. It is most commonly seen in the head and neck region (40%) and in the genital region (25%). Other areas of involvement are the thorax, abdomen, and extremities. On US, they appear as hypoechoic and heterogeneous masses with increased vascularity on Doppler examination. On MRI, they demonstrate intermediate signal on T1-weighted images, high signal on T2-weighted images, and marked enhancement after gadolin-ium injection [64]. Embryonal rhabdomyosarco-mas tend to be more homogeneous, while alveolar and pleomorphic rhabdomyosarcomas are more heterogeneous and often contain necrosis. While restricted diffusion is observed in solid areas, no restriction is seen in the areas of necrosis or bleeding. In addition, dynamic contrast-enhanced MRI demonstrates a type 3 or 4 enhancement pattern in solid areas and a type 1 enhancement pattern in areas of necrosis or bleeding [65].

3.5.6 Malignant Nerve Sheath Tumors

Malignant nerve sheath tumors represent 5–10% of all malignant soft tissue tumors and are seen in the age range of 20–50 years [66]. More than half of the cases are seen together with neurofibroma-tosis type 1. It often involves major nerves such as the sciatic nerve, brachial nerve, and sacral plexus. Imaging features are similar to other nerve sheath tumors. However, tumors larger than 5 cm, heterogeneous appearance due to necrosis and hemorrhage, irregular margins, presence of peritumoral edema, rapid and hetero-geneous contrast enhancement, destruction of adjacent bone structures, and presence of regional lymphadenopathy are findings suggesting malig-nancy. On US, they appear as heterogeneous hypoechoic fusiform masses associated with the peripheral nerve, containing a pseudocapsule representing a partially and irregularly thickened

hyperechoic nerve sheath [67]. On MRI, they appear as a mass with irregular borders, larger than 5 cm, infiltrating the surrounding tissues. In addition, heterogeneity, central necrosis, and peripheral nodular heterogeneous enhancement may be seen [68].

3.5.7 Undifferentiated Pleomorphic Sarcoma

Undifferentiated pleomorphic sarcoma occurs most commonly in the lower extremity, and less frequently in the upper extremity [69]. It is the most common soft tissue sarcoma after radiother-apy [8]. On US examination, it has a large size, heterogeneous echotexture, hypoechoic and infil-trative appearance with irregular borders, and often has increased vascularity [8, 30]. They may be very large and may present with destructive findings in the adjacent bone [70]. On US, they are seen as hypoechoic masses with central necrosis or calcification and irregular margins. Doppler US demonstrates vascularization in solid parts [71]. Variable findings are seen on MRI depending on cellularity, myxoid content, bleeding, necrosis, and calcification. Peripheral contrast enhancement is frequently observed because of hemorrhage, necrosis, and myxoid content in the central part of the tumor.

3.5.8 Soft Tissue Metastases and Lymphoma

Lung, kidney, and colon cancers are the most common malignancies that metastasize to soft tissue. The most common sites of metastasis are the thigh muscles, iliopsoas, and paravertebral muscles [72]. On US examination, soft tissue metastases appear as hypoechoic masses with increased vascularity and infiltrative margins [30]. Destructive changes and fragmentation in the adjacent bones can be seen and it may repre-sent the extension of the bone lesion into the adjacent soft tissue or vice versa. Posterior acous-tic enhancement may be seen in some lesions. Associated hyperemia is typically present [70].

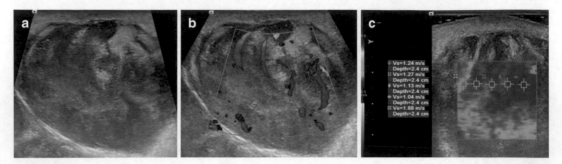

Fig. 3.6 A 67-year-old woman with a soft tissue mass in her left thigh. The mass is located superficial to the fascia, 12 cm in its largest dimension, hypoechoic and heterogeneous in echotexture (**a**). Doppler US examination demonstrates central and peripheral vascularity (**b**). SWE examination and SWV measurements of the lesion are demonstrated (**c**). Histopathological examination revealed a lymphoma of the soft tissue

On MRI, soft tissue metastases are observed as poorly circumscribed lesions with low signal on T1-weighted images, and high signal on T2-weighted images [73]. Extensive peritumoral enhancement with central necrosis is a common finding [74].

Primary soft tissue lymphoma is very rare. It is usually seen in patients over 60 years of age. Patients clinically present with an intramuscular mass [75]. Most soft tissue lymphomas occur in the trunk and lower extremities. Soft tissue lymphomas are seen as homogenous hypoechoic lesions with infiltrating margins [76]. Posterior acoustic enhancement may be seen. On Doppler US, the tumor demonstrates increased vascularity (Fig. 3.6). On MRI, they appear homogeneously isointense or slightly hypointense on T1-weighted images and hyperintense on T2-weighted images. They demonstrate homogeneous enhancement after contrast material administration [77].

3.6 Conclusion and Future Perspectives

Elastography is a recently developed US-based imaging method that allows the evaluation of tissue elasticity during US examination. In this chapter, we summarized the current literature on US and elastography in the diagnosis of malignant soft tissue tumors. While elastography was found to be effective in the diagnosis of malignant soft tissue tumors in some studies, its diagnostic efficacy could not be demonstrated in other studies. In most of these studies, the study population consisted of a wide variety of tumor subtypes. Soft tissue tumors can contain a wide variety of cell types such as calcification, fibrotic changes, hemorrhage, necrosis, and cystic degeneration. Since soft tissue tumors contain such heterogeneous histological tissues, different results have been obtained in studies in the literature. This may explain the limitation of elasticity measurement in the differentiation of malignant and benign soft tissue tumors. Based on the current literature, it is obvious that more studies with larger patient populations are needed on this subject. Considering the foregoing, someone may think to investigate the efficacy of elastography in differentiating tumors with similar histological features (e.g., differentiation of malignant fibroblastic tumors and benign fibroblastic tumors). However, since the histological subtype of the tumor cannot be known at the stage of US examination in a patient presenting with a soft tissue tumor, it may be clinically difficult to evaluate the efficacy of US elastography in the diagnosis of malignant lesions in a particular histological subtype, and its contribution to the clinical practice may be questionable. It seems that MRI will likely continue to be an invaluable imaging method in the diagnosis of malignant soft tissue tumors, as it provides important information about various histological components of the tumors such as fat, fibrotic tissue, hemorrhage, and necrosis, thanks to its high soft tissue resolution and different signal properties in T1 and T2 sequences. The diagnostic performance of conventional US has also been proven to be effective in differentiating malignant and benign lesions. Thanks to conventional US findings, a significant portion of malignant lesions can be diagnosed with the US. Considering all this information, future studies with larger populations may also focus on the contribution of elastography to MRI and conventional US findings, besides investigating the diagnostic efficacy of elastography alone.

References

1. Andritsch E, Beishon M, Bielack S, Bonvalot S, Casali P, Crul M, et al. ECCO essential requirements for quality cancer care: soft tissue sarcoma in adults and bone sarcoma. A critical review. Crit Rev Oncol Hematol. 2017;110:94–105. https://doi.org/10.1016/J.CRITREVONC.2016.12.002.
2. Noebauer-Huhmann IM, Weber MA, Lalam RK, Trattnig S, Bohndorf K, Vanhoenacker F, et al. Soft tissue tumors in adults: ESSR-approved guidelines for diagnostic imaging. Semin Musculoskelet Radiol. 2015;19:475–82. https://doi.org/10.1055/S-0035-1569251/ID/JR00863-49.
3. Ozturk M, Polat AV, Selcuk MB. Whole-lesion ADC histogram analysis versus single-slice ADC measurement for the differentiation of benign and malignant soft tissue tumors. Eur J Radiol. 2021;143:109934. https://doi.org/10.1016/J.EJRAD.2021.109934.
4. Ozturk M, Polat AV, Tosun FC, Selcuk MB. Does the SUVmax of FDG-PET/CT correlate with the ADC values of DWI in musculoskeletal malignancies? J Belgian Soc Radiol. 2021;105:11. https://doi.org/10.5334/JBSR.2378.
5. Hicks RJ. Functional imaging techniques for evaluation of sarcomas. Cancer Imaging. 2005;5:58. https://doi.org/10.1102/1470-7330.2005.0007.
6. Katal S, Gholamrezanezhad A, Kessler M, Olyaei M, Jadvar H. PET in the diagnostic management of soft tissue sarcomas of musculoskeletal origin. PET Clin. 2018;13:609–21. https://doi.org/10.1016/J.CPET.2018.05.011.
7. Bruno F, Arrigoni F, Mariani S, Splendiani A, Di Cesare E, Masciocchi C, et al. Advanced magnetic resonance imaging (MRI) of soft tissue tumors: techniques and applications. Radiol Med. 2019;124:243–52. https://doi.org/10.1007/S11547-019-01035-7/FIGURES/4.
8. Aparisi Gómez MP, Errani C, Lalam R, Vasilevska Nikodinovska V, Fanti S, Tagliafico AS, et al. The role of ultrasound in the diagnosis of soft tissue tumors.

9. Semin Musculoskelet Radiol. 2020;24:135–55. https://doi.org/10.1055/S-0039-3402060.
9. Gürüf A, Öztürk M, Bayrak İK, Polat AV. Shear wave versus strain elastography in the differentiation of benign and malignant breast lesions. Turkish J Med Sci. 2019;49:1509–17. https://doi.org/10.3906/SAG-1905-15.
10. Turgut E, Celenk C, Tanrivermis Sayit A, Bekci T, Gunbey HP, Aslan K. Efficiency of B-mode ultrasound and strain elastography in differentiating between benign and malignant cervical lymph nodes. Ultrasound Q. 2017;33:201–7. https://doi.org/10.1097/RUQ.0000000000000302.
11. Gürün E, Akdulum İ, Akyüz M, Oktar SÖ. Shear wave elastography evaluation of brachial plexus in multiple sclerosis. Acta Radiol. 2022;63:520–6. https://doi.org/10.1177/02841851211002828.
12. Gurun E, Akdulum I, Akyuz M, Tokgoz N, Ozhan Oktar S. Shear wave elastography evaluation of meniscus degeneration with magnetic resonance imaging correlation. Acad Radiol. 2021;28:1383–8. https://doi.org/10.1016/J.ACRA.2020.12.013.
13. Aslan S, Ceyhan Bilgici M, Saglam D, Ozturk M. The role of ARFI elastography to evaluate microstructural changes of patients with testicular microlithiasis. Acta Radiol. 2018;59:1517–22. https://doi.org/10.1177/0284185118764213.
14. Berg WA, Cosgrove DO, Doré CJ, Schäfer FKW, Svensson WE, Hooley RJ, et al. Shear-wave elastography improves the specificity of breast US: the BE1 multinational study of 939 masses. Radiology. 2012;262:435–49. https://doi.org/10.1148/RADIOL.11110640.
15. Lu Q, Ling W, Lu C, Li J, Ma L, Quan J, et al. Hepatocellular carcinoma: stiffness value and ratio to discriminate malignant from benign focal liver lesions. Radiology. 2015;275:880–8. https://doi.org/10.1148/RADIOL.14131164.
16. Lyshchik A, Higashi T, Asato R, Tanaka S, Ito J, Mal JJ, et al. Thyroid gland tumor diagnosis at US elastography. Radiology. 2005;237:202–11. https://doi.org/10.1148/RADIOL.2363041248.
17. Hahn S, Lee YH, Lee SH, Suh JS. Value of the strain ratio on ultrasonic elastography for differentiation of benign and malignant soft tissue tumors. J Ultrasound Med. 2017;36:121–7. https://doi.org/10.7863/ultra.16.01054.
18. Pass B, Jafari M, Rowbotham E, Hensor EMA, Gupta H, Robinson P. Do quantitative and qualitative shear wave elastography have a role in evaluating musculoskeletal soft tissue masses? Eur Radiol. 2017;27:723–31. https://doi.org/10.1007/s00330-016-4427-y.
19. Pass B, Johnson M, Hensor EMA, Gupta H, Robinson P. Sonoelastography of musculoskeletal soft tissue masses: a pilot study of quantitative evaluation. J Ultrasound Med. 2016;35:2209–16. https://doi.org/10.7863/ultra.15.11065.
20. Riishede I, Ewertsen C, Carlsen J, Petersen MM, Jensen F, Nielsen MB. Strain elastography for prediction of malignancy in soft tissue tumours—pre-

liminary results. Ultraschall Med. 2015;36:369–74. https://doi.org/10.1055/S-0034-1399289.

21. Ozturk M, Selcuk MB, Polat AV, Ozbalci AB, Baris YS. The diagnostic value of ultrasound and shear wave elastography in the differentiation of benign and malignant soft tissue tumors. Skeletal Radiol. 2020;49:1795–805. https://doi.org/10.1007/s00256-020-03492-y.

22. Dou Y, Xuan J, Zhao T, Li X, Wang H, Zhang Y, et al. The diagnostic performance of conventional ultrasound and strain elastography in malignant soft tissue tumors. Skeletal Radiol. 2021;50:1677–86. https://doi.org/10.1007/S00256-021-03724-9.

23. Ohshika S, Saruga T, Ogawa T, Ono H, Ishibashi Y. Distinction between benign and malignant soft tissue tumors based on an ultrasonographic evaluation of vascularity and elasticity. Oncol Lett. 2021;21:281. https://doi.org/10.3892/OL.2021.12542.

24. Li S, Liu L, Lv G. Diagnostic value of strain elastography for differentiating benign and malignant soft tissue masses. Oncol Lett. 2017;14:2041–4. https://doi.org/10.3892/OL.2017.6385.

25. Nicholls J, Alfuraih AM, Hensor EMA, Robinson P. Inter- and intra-reader reproducibility of shear wave elastography measurements for musculoskeletal soft tissue masses. Skeletal Radiol. 2020;49:779–86. https://doi.org/10.1007/S00256-019-03300-2.

26. Winn N, Baldwin J, Cassar-Pullicino V, Cool P, Ockendon M, Tins B, et al. Characterization of soft tissue tumours with ultrasound, shear wave elastography and MRI. Skeletal Radiol. 2020;49:869–81. https://doi.org/10.1007/S00256-019-03363-1.

27. Kransdorf MJ, Murphey MD, Wessell DE, Cassidy RC, Czuczman GJ, Demertzis JL, et al. ACR appropriateness criteria ® soft-tissue masses. J Am Coll Radiol. 2018;15:S189–97. https://doi.org/10.1016/j.jacr.2018.03.012.

28. Lakkaraju A, Sinha R, Garikipati R, Edward S, Robinson P. Ultrasound for initial evaluation and triage of clinically suspicious soft-tissue masses. Clin Radiol. 2009;64:615–21. https://doi.org/10.1016/J.CRAD.2009.01.012.

29. Datir A, James SLJ, Ali K, Lee J, Ahmad M, Saifuddin A. MRI of soft-tissue masses: the relationship between lesion size, depth, and diagnosis. Clin Radiol. 2008;63:373–8. https://doi.org/10.1016/j.crad.2007.08.016.

30. Taljanovic MS, Gimber LH, Klauser AS, Porrino JA, Chadaz TS, Omar IM. Ultrasound in the evaluation of musculoskeletal soft-tissue masses. Semin Roentgenol. 2017;52:241–54. https://doi.org/10.1053/j.ro.2017.08.002.

31. Pierucci A, Teixeira P, Zimmermann V, Sirveaux F, Rios M, Verhaegue JL, et al. Tumours and pseudotumours of the soft tissue in adults: perspectives and current role of sonography. Diagn Interv Imaging. 2013;94:238–54. https://doi.org/10.1016/J.DIII.2012.10.018.

32. Di Domenico P, Middleton W. Sonographic evaluation of palpable superficial masses. Radiol Clin North

Am. 2014;52:1295–305. https://doi.org/10.1016/j.rcl.2014.07.011.

33. Li A, Peng XJ, Ma Q, Dong Y, Mao CL, Hu Y. Diagnostic performance of conventional ultrasound and quantitative and qualitative real-time shear wave elastography in musculoskeletal soft tissue tumors. J Orthop Surg Res. 2020;15:103. https://doi.org/10.1186/S13018-020-01620-X.

34. Tavare AN, Alfuraih AM, Hensor EMA, Astrinakis E, Gupta H, Robinson P. Shear-wave elastography of benign versus malignant musculoskeletal soft-tissue masses: comparison with conventional US and MRI. Radiology. 2019;290:410–7. https://doi.org/10.1148/radiol.2018180950.

35. Morii T, Kishino T, Shimamori N, Motohashi M, Ohnishi H, Honya K, et al. Differential diagnosis between benign and malignant soft tissue tumors utilizing ultrasound parameters. J Med Ultrason. 2018;45:113–9. https://doi.org/10.1007/s10396-017-0796-3.

36. Carra BJ, Bui-Mansfield LT, O'Brien SD, Chen DC. Sonography of musculoskeletal soft-tissue masses: techniques, pearls, and pitfalls. Am J Roentgenol. 2014;202:1281–90. https://doi.org/10.2214/AJR.13.11564.

37. Giovagnorio F, Andreoli C, De Cicco ML. Color Doppler sonography of focal lesions of the skin and subcutaneous tissue. J Ultrasound Med. 1999;18:89–93. https://doi.org/10.7863/JUM.1999.18.2.89.

38. Catalano O, Varelli C, Sbordone C, Corvino A, De Rosa D, Vallone G, et al. A bump: what to do next? Ultrasound imaging of superficial soft-tissue palpable lesions. J Ultrasound. 2020;23:287. https://doi.org/10.1007/S40477-019-00415-Z.

39. Sigrist RMS, Liau J, El Kaffas A, Chammas MC, Willmann JK. Ultrasound elastography: review of techniques and clinical applications. Theranostics. 2017;7:1303–29. https://doi.org/10.7150/THNO.18650.

40. Bamber J, Cosgrove D, Dietrich CF, Fromageau J, Bojunga J, Calliada F, et al. EFSUMB guidelines and recommendations on the clinical use of ultrasound elastographypart 1: basic principles and technology. Ultraschall Der Medizin. 2013;34:169–84. https://doi.org/10.1055/s-0033-1335205.

41. Klauser AS, Miyamoto H, Bellmann-Weiler R, Feuchtner GM, Wick MC, Jaschke WR. Sonoelastography: musculoskeletal applications. Radiology. 2014;272:622–33. https://doi.org/10.1148/RADIOL.14121765.

42. Park HJ, Lee SY, Lee SM, Kim WT, Lee S, Ahn KS. Strain elastography features of epidermoid tumours in superficial soft tissue: differences from other benign soft-tissue tumours and malignant tumours. Br J Radiol. 2015;88:20140797. https://doi.org/10.1259/bjr.20140797.

43. Itoh A, Ueno E, Tohno E, Kamma H, Takahashi H, Shiina T, et al. Breast disease: clinical application of US elastography for diagnosis. Radiology. 2006;239:341–50. https://doi.org/10.1148/RADIOL.2391041676.

44. Cohen J, Riishede I, Carlsen JF, Lambine TL, Dam MS, Petersen MM, et al. Can strain elastography predict malignancy of soft tissue tumors in a tertiary sarcoma center? Diagnostics. 2020;10:148. https://doi.org/10.3390/DIAGNOSTICS10030148.

45. Magarelli N, Carducci C, Bucalo C, Filograna L, Rapisarda S, De Waure C, et al. Sonoelastography for qualitative and quantitative evaluation of superficial soft tissue lesions: a feasibility study. Eur Radiol. 2014;24:566–73. https://doi.org/10.1007/s00330-013-3069-6.

46. Lalitha P, Balaji Reddy M, Jagannath RK. Musculoskeletal applications of elastography: a pictorial essay of our initial experience. Korean J Radiol. 2011;12:365–75. https://doi.org/10.3348/KJR.2011.12.3.365.

47. Scaperrotta G, Ferranti C, Costa C, Mariani L, Marchesini M, Suman L, et al. Role of sonoelastography in non-palpable breast lesions. Eur Radiol. 2008;18:2381–9. https://doi.org/10.1007/S00330-008-1032-8.

48. Ophir J, Alam SK, Garra BS, Kallel F, Konofagou EE, Krouskop T, et al. Elastography: imaging the elastic properties of soft tissues with ultrasound. J Med Ultrason. 2001;2002(29):155–71. https://doi.org/10.1007/BF02480847.

49. Bansal A, Goyal S, Goyal A, Jana M. WHO classification of soft tissue tumours 2020: an update and simplified approach for radiologists. Eur J Radiol. 2021;143:109937. https://doi.org/10.1016/J.EJRAD.2021.109937.

50. Wagner JM, Rebik K, Spicer PJ. Ultrasound of soft tissue masses and fluid collections. Radiol Clin North Am. 2019;57:657–69. https://doi.org/10.1016/J.RCL.2019.01.013.

51. Fenzl L, Mehrmann M, Kremp K, Schneider G. Soft tissue tumors: Epidemiology, classification and staging. Radiologe. 2017;57:973–86. https://doi.org/10.1007/S00117-017-0320-1.

52. Murphey MD, Smith WS, Smith SE, Kransdorf MJ, Temple HT. From the archives of the AFIP: imaging of musculoskeletal neurogenic tumors—radiologic-pathologic correlation. Radiographics. 1999;19:1253–80.https://doi.org/10.1148/radiographics.19.5.g99se101253.

53. Gupta P, Potti TA, Wuertzer SD, Lenchik L, Pacholke DA. Spectrum of fat-containing soft-tissue masses at MR imaging: the common, the uncommon, the characteristic, and the sometimes confusing. Radiographics. 2016;36:753–66. https://doi.org/10.1148/RG.2016150133.

54. Shen Y, Ren Y, Wang W, Wang Y, Yang Y, Wu F, et al. Solitary fibrous tumor of the spine: imaging grading diagnosis and prognosis. J Comput Assist Tomogr. 2022;46:638–44. https://doi.org/10.1097/RCT.0000000000001319.

55. Shanbhogue AK, Prasad SR, Takahashi N, Vikram R, Zaheer A, Sandrasegaran K. Somatic and visceral solitary fibrous tumors in the abdomen and pelvis: cross-sectional imaging spectrum. Radiographics.

2011;31:393–408. https://doi.org/10.1148/RG.312105080.

56. Wat SYJ, Sur M, Dhamanaskar K. Solitary fibrous tumor (SFT) of the pelvis. Clin Imaging. 2008;32:152–6. https://doi.org/10.1016/J.CLINIMAG.2007.07.003.

57. Hourani R, Taslakian B, Shabb NS, Nassar L, Hourani MH, Moukarbel R, et al. Fibroblastic and myofibroblastic tumors of the head and neck: comprehensive imaging-based review with pathologic correlation. Eur J Radiol. 2015;84:250–60. https://doi.org/10.1016/j.ejrad.2014.10.017.

58. Morag Y, Lucas DR. Ultrasound of myxofibrosarcoma. Skeletal Radiol. 2022;51:691–700. https://doi.org/10.1007/S00256-021-03869-7.

59. Hwang S, Kelliher E, Hameed M. Imaging features of low-grade fibromyxoid sarcoma (Evans tumor). Skeletal Radiol. 2012;41:1263–72. https://doi.org/10.1007/S00256-012-1417-2.

60. Wiegand S, Dietz A, Wichmann G. Malignant vascular tumors of the head and neck-which type of therapy works best? Cancers (Basel). 2021;13:6201. https://doi.org/10.3390/CANCERS13246201.

61. Razek AA, Huang BY. Soft tissue tumors of the head and neck: imaging-based review of the WHO classification. Radiographics. 2011;31:1923–54. https://doi.org/10.1148/RG.317115095.

62. Ostlere SJ. Ultrasound of soft tissue masses. In: McNally E, editor. Practical musculoskeletal ultrasound. London: Elsevier; 2014. p. 387–407.

63. Rha SE, Byun JY, Jung SE, Lee SL, Cho SM, Hwang SS, et al. CT and MRI of uterine sarcomas and their mimickers. AJR Am J Roentgenol. 2003;181:1369–74. https://doi.org/10.2214/AJR.181.5.1811369.

64. Van Rijn RR, Wilde JCH, Bras J, Oldenburger F, McHugh KMC, Merks JHM. Imaging findings in non-craniofacial childhood rhabdomyosarcoma. Pediatr Radiol. 2008;38:617–34. https://doi.org/10.1007/S00247-008-0751-Y.

65. Clemente EJI, Navallas M, de la Torre IBM, Suñol M, Del Cerro JM, Torner F, et al. MRI of rhabdomyosarcoma and other soft-tissue sarcomas in children. Radiographics. 2020;40:791–814. https://doi.org/10.1148/RG.2020190119/ASSET/IMAGES/LARGE/RG.2020190119.FIG14A.JPEG.

66. Selçuk MB, Polat AV. Yumuşak doku tümörleri: radyolojik özellikler. In: Dabak N, editor. Multidisipliner Yaklaşımla Kem. ve Yumuşak Doku Tümörleri. 2nd ed. Ankara; 2017.

67. Rafailidis V, Kaziani T, Theocharides C, Papanikolaou A, Rafailidis D. Imaging of the malignant peripheral nerve sheath tumour with emphasis on ultrasonography: correlation with MRI. J Ultrasound. 2014;17:219. https://doi.org/10.1007/S40477-014-0097-2.

68. Lin J, Martel W. Cross-sectional imaging of peripheral nerve sheath tumors: characteristic signs on CT, MR imaging, and sonography. AJR Am J Roentgenol. 2001;176:75–82. https://doi.org/10.2214/AJR.176.1.1760075.

69. Kumar V, Abbas A, Fausto N, Robbins S, Cotran R, editors. Robbins and Cotran pathologic basis of dis-

ease. 7th ed. Elsevier Saunders: Philadelphia, PA; 2015.

70. Chiou HJ, Chou YH, Chiu SY, Wang HK, Chen WM, Chen TH, et al. Differentiation of benign and malignant superficial soft-tissue masses using gray-scale and color Doppler ultrasonography. J Chin Med Assoc. 2009;72:307–15. https://doi.org/10.1016/S1726-4901(09)70377-6.

71. Reddy R. Primary undifferentiated pleomorphic sarcoma of the biceps femoris muscle compli-cated by hemorrhage: an underrecognized entity. Cureus. 2021;13:e16958. https://doi.org/10.7759/CUREUS.16958.

72. Gielen J, Vanhoenacker FM, Ceulemans R, Van Holsbeeck M, Van der Woude HJ, Verstraete KL, et al. Ultrasound and color Doppler ultrasound of soft tissue tumors and tumorlike lesions. In: Imaging soft tissue tumors. Berlin: Springer International Publishing; 2017. p. 3–40. https://doi.org/10.1007/978-3-319-46679-8_1/COVER.

73. Perisano C, Spinelli MS, Graci C, Scaramuzzo L, Marzetti E, Barone C, et al. Soft tissue metastases in lung cancer: a review of the literature. Eur Rev Med Pharmacol Sci. 2012;16:1908–14.

74. Tuoheti Y, Okada K, Osanai T, Nishida J, Ehara S, Hashimoto M, et al. Skeletal muscle metastases of car-cinoma: a clinicopathological study of 12 cases. Jpn J Clin Oncol. 2004;34:210–4. https://doi.org/10.1093/JJCO/HYH036.

75. Ozturk M, Cinka H, Polat AV, Say F, Selcuk MB. Primary muscle lymphoma in an elderly patient: ultrasound and magnetic resonance imaging find-ings. Am J Diagn Imaging. 2019;5:1–3. https://doi.org/10.5455/ajdi.20181001021931.

76. Chiou HJ, Chou YH, Chiou SY, Chen WM, Chen W, Wan HK, et al. Superficial soft-tissue lym-phoma: sonographic appearance and early survival. Ultrasound Med Biol. 2006;32:1287–97. https://doi.org/10.1016/J.ULTRASMEDBIO.2006.05.011.

77. Ruzek KA, Wenger DE. The multiple faces of lym-phoma of the musculoskeletal system. Skeletal Radiol. 2004;33:1–8. https://doi.org/10.1007/S00256-003-0709-Y.

Tendons and Ligaments

4

Domenico Albano, Mariachiara Basile,
Salvatore Gitto, Francesca Serpi,
Carmelo Messina, and Luca Maria Sconfienza

4.1 Introduction

Over the last years, sonoelastography has been increasingly used as an imaging tool able to help in evaluating tendons and ligaments status and composition, from both a quantitative and qualitative point of view, in addition to the conventional B-mode ultrasound imaging [1]. Two sonoelastography methods are commonly used in musculoskeletal research and clinical practice: strain elastography (SE), in which a mechanical force compresses the tissues axially, and shear-wave elastography (SWE), in which compressive acoustic waves dynamically provide local stress in the soft tissues [2].

SE is the original form of elastography, it requires the application of an external compressive force exerted by the operator or internal forces generated by pulsatile structures within the body to cause tissue deformation. SE enables to assess the deformation of the soft tissues along the propagation axis of the beam through the analysis of the RF signal along each line of scanning. The resulting color elastogram that is generated is overlaid on the B-mode gray-scale image. This color map provides the operator with qualitative information about the tissue elasticity that varies according to specific colors. The stiffness of tendons and ligaments may therefore be evaluated qualitatively and should be interpreted on the basis of the displayed color bar given that some users prefer the red color to depict stiffer tendons/ligaments and the blue color for softer structures and vice versa. It should be considered that only pseudo-quantitative information can be obtained from SE by calculating strain ratios that can be used to compare the target tissue strain with that of closing healthy tissue, with a strain ratio > 1 indicating a stiffer target tissue. A "spacer" between the US probe and the skin can be used to convey more homogeneous pressure, thereby reducing artifacts [3].

SWE allows for a quantitative and reproducible approach for evaluating the stiffness of tendons and ligaments, being less operator-dependent than SE [4–6]. A focused acoustic radiation force is delivered from a linear US probe to induce shear waves throughout the soft tissues. These shear waves propagate perpen-

D. Albano
IRCCS Istituto Ortopedico Galeazzi, Milan, Italy

M. Basile
Scuola di Specializzazione in Radiodiagnostica,
Università degli Studi di Milano, Milan, Italy

S. Gitto · F. Serpi
Dipartimento di Scienze Biomediche per la Salute,
Università degli Studi di Milano, Milan, Italy

C. Messina · L. M. Sconfienza (✉)
IRCCS Istituto Ortopedico Galeazzi, Milan, Italy

Dipartimento di Scienze Biomediche per la Salute,
Università degli Studi di Milano, Milan, Italy
e-mail: io@lucasconfienza.it

dicularly at a slower velocity than the US beam, resulting in particle displacements that can be calculated using a speckle tracking algorithm. Tissue displacement maps are used to measure shear wave velocity expressed in meters per second. The distribution of shear wave velocities at each pixel is directly related to the shear modulus G (ratio of stress to strain) which is calculated by a simple mathematical equation and expresses the tissue stiffness and elasticity in units of pressure, usually kilopascals. Because soft tissues with small deformations are usually assumed to be incompressible, G is sometimes converted to the Young modulus E by the simple eq. $E = 3G$ for incompressible media. In SWE, as in SE, a color-coded elastogram can be overlaid on the B-mode US with specific colors indicating softer or stiffer tendons and ligaments. These colors are determined by the speed of propagation of the shear waves through the tendon and ligament fibers. Red color generally corresponds to stiffer structures, while blue to softer ones, with green and yellow being associated with moderately elastic tendons and ligaments. In contrast to SE, SWE allows for quantitative measurements from any portion of the investigated tendon/ligament within the color elastogram due to the sequencing of particle displacements made possible by ultrafast analysis [1].

Tendons and ligaments have, in normal conditions, a characteristic elasticity coefficient due to their intrinsic mechanical properties, which can undergo changes in pathological conditions. Sonoelastography can be indicated when the ultrasound examination is not conclusive, since healthy tendon and ligament fibers can present the same echotexture on ultrasound B-mode images, showing different elasticity on ES images [7, 8]. During the past years, several studies have been published on the application of ES on tendons and ligaments with promising results. Specifically, there are just international recommendations that, based on strong evidence, suggest the use of sonoelastography on some tendons, while fewer indications have been established on ligamentous structures [9].

4.2 Tendons

Tendon-related pathologies, such as tendinopathy, are associated with professional sports, and some working activities, but are also observed in general population. Generally, the diagnostic work-up includes clinical evaluation and imaging examinations, mostly using ultrasound as a first-level imaging modality, followed by magnetic resonance [10]. Additionally, the assessment of the elastic properties of soft tissues, provided by sonoelastography, has proven to be valuable in identifying pathologic conditions involving the tendons [11]. ES can be especially important for evaluating tendon status given that mild tendinopathies do not determine substantial changes in ultrasound echotexture and especially in magnetic resonance signals of tendon fibers [12]. Repetitive microtrauma, overload, and vascular alterations cause tissue damage that impact on the elasticity of the fibrillary architecture [5]. As a matter of fact, degenerative changes include an increase in collagen type III fibers, and fibrocartilaginous changes thereby decreasing the stiffness of pathologic tendons [13].

4.2.1 Achilles Tendon

Achilles tendinopathy is generally assessed by ultrasound, evaluating thickness, echotexture in B-mode, and vascularization through power Doppler [14, 15]. Further, several authors used sonoelastography to evaluate the stiffness of normal and pathologic Achilles tendons in different postures, highlighting the importance of both spatial location of sonoelastography assessment and ankle posture for the evaluation of the tendon viscoelastic properties [16]. The Achilles tendon is the strongest and thickest tendon in the human body, has a superficial location, and is well differentiated from surrounding tissues, making it particularly suitable for sonoelastography assessment [17]. Healthy Achilles tendons have a homogeneous and stiff elastosonographic pattern that is prevalently red in SE images, expressing a certain rigidity and scarce deformability, with high SWE velocities values

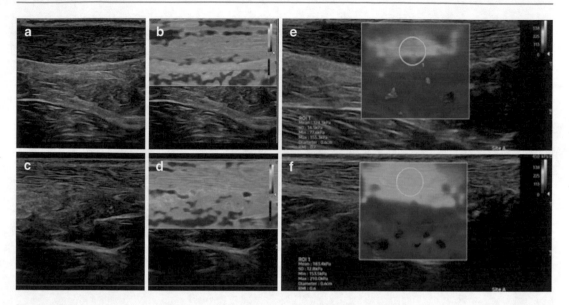

Fig. 4.1 US images of a patient with non-insertional Achilles tendinopathy showing a thickened and hypoechoic tendon on B-mode (**a**) and heterogeneous elastogram (**b**) with regions of yellow and red coloring corresponding to tendon softening. US of a healthy sub-ject with normal Achilles tendon on B-mode (**c**) and a homogeneous elastogram (**d**). Also note the different stiffness values of the pathologic (**e**, mean = 124 kPa) and normal (**f**, mean = 183 kPa) Achilles tendons on SWE

that exceed 300 kPa [1]. Studies of Achilles tendons conducted on athletes revealed higher stiffness in frequent exercisers than in infrequent exercisers and demonstrated that tendon softening may predict pain and tendinopathy providing time for early intervention [18, 19]. Other authors described that low Achilles SWE velocity is associated with higher age, self-reported pain and disability, and decreased loading capacity of the Achilles tendon [20], while no significant differences depending on sex were identified.

In agreement with the most recent literature, the VISA-A (Victorian Institute of Sport Assessment-Achilles questionnaire) scale showed a weak correlation with standard ultrasound and power Doppler characteristics, but that was strongly correlated with the elasticity values ($p = 0.0001$, df = 83, $\tau\beta = 0.71$). Sensitivity for standard ultrasound alone and standard ultrasound plus SWE for asymptomatic tendons was 0.58 and 0.78, respectively. Hence, the use of SWE revealed high specificity in the detection of tendinopathy, particularly subclinical tendinopathy, increasing the diagnostic performance of conventional ultrasound for Achilles tendinopathy (Fig. 4.1) [21, 22].

Subclinical changes of the Achilles tendon were also shown with sonoelastography in patients with ankylosing spondylitis, acromegaly, and in patients with diabetic ulcers [17]. In case of tendon rupture, the Achilles tendon is seen as blue or turquoise in the ES images, since the loss of tension and the presence of hematoma or effusion contribute to a significant reduction in stiffness with a mean velocity less or equal to 4.06 m/s and signal-void areas at SWE [23, 24]. ES utility was also investigated after surgical repair of Achilles tendon rupture. After surgery, there is an increased tendon stiffness and heterogeneity according to the physiological healing process, likely due to the structural alteration of collagen fibers, with a predominance of type III collagen instead of type I. SWE results showed that repaired tendons gradually became stiffer postoperatively. In a previous paper, the mean values of elastic modulus of the repaired tendons were respectively 187.7 kPa at 12 weeks, 238.3 kPa at 24 weeks, and 289.6 kPa at 48 weeks. Likely, the mean AOFAS (American Orthopaedic Foot &

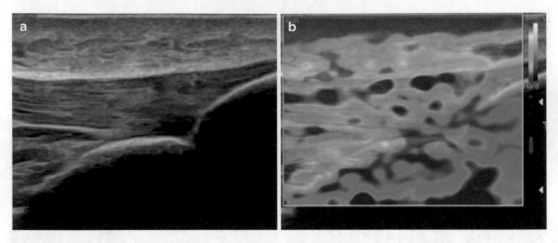

Fig. 4.2 Patellar tendinopathy of a runner with US B-mode just showing slightly hypoechoic distal fibers (**a**), with heterogeneous elastogram (**b**)

Ankle Society) scores were significantly different among the three postoperative time points. Elasticity was significantly and positively correlated with the AOFAS scores (P = 0.0003, OR = 0.9159) [25, 26]. An increased consistency was also reported in the contralateral tendon [19], probably due to overload during the rehabilitation [25]. A positive correlation between the degree of tendon functionality and its elasticity was found, suggesting that increased stiffness and lower elastic modulus values might predict poor mechanical properties, and functional outcomes, with worse healing of repaired tendons [26].

Therefore, sonoelastography improves the performance of ultrasound for Achilles tendinopathy, particularly increasing the capability of detecting of subtle changes in the tendon (Fig. 4.1).

4.2.2 Patellar Tendon

Patellar tendinopathy is an overuse injury of the patellar tendon, prevalent in athletes, resulting in pain and impaired function [27]. Patellar tendinopathy is characterized by disruption and disorganization of the tendon fibers, along with an increase in tendon thickness, structural abnormalities, alterations of the tendon's mechanical properties and of the function of the knee joint [13, 14]. Conventional ultrasound shows

hypoechoic areas within the tendon. However, ultrasound changes can be subtle or absent, while asymptomatic subjects may present abnormal tendon morphology at ultrasound, including hypoechogenic changes [28, 29].

Therefore, sonoelastography may offer an independent and complementary approach to the acoustic impedance and vascular flow information provided by B-mode and Doppler imaging. Studies using SE and SWE concerning elasticity characterization of patellar tendinopathy had discrepant results. Some described a decrease in stiffness (Fig. 4.2) [30–32] and others, using SWE, documented a higher shear elastic modulus and, therefore, increased stiffness in patellar tendinopathy [20, 33]. The soft pattern at SE of healthy patellar tendons may be explained by the fact that the patellar tendon is connected to two hard and fixed structures, patellar bone, and tibial tuberosity, contrary to the other investigated tendons, connected on one side to a muscle [34].

A study assessing athletes with unilateral patellar tendinopathy using SWE found a correlation between increased stiffness of the tendon and the intensity of pain and degree of dysfunction. The mean shear elastic modulus in the painful side was 43.6 kPa, while in the non-painful side it was significantly lower (25.8 kPa; p = 0.008) [33]. Using SE, another study described symptomatic patellar tendons in athletes as softer than asymptomatic ones and showed that sonoelastography increased conventional ultrasound sensitivity (72.5%) and accuracy (60%) in the diagnosis of patellar tendinopathy allowing a better correlation to functional scores [32].

Hence, it is still unclear which pattern and elasticity values can differentiate healthy from pathologic patellar tendons. Methodological differences, such as ultrasound equipment and sample size, can partly explain these incongruences. Moreover, it seems that SWE may depict tendon healing better than B-mode ultrasound helping in monitoring treatment effects. The thickness of patellar tendons decreases after treatment, generally not returning to normal levels. Likely, athletes with patellar tendinopathy showing higher elastic modulus see a decrease after treatment, with a strong negative correlation between the elastic modulus and VISA-P scores at the different follow-up sessions [$r = -0.784$, $P < 0.001$ (1 month); $r = 0.877$, $P < 0.001$ (3 months)]. The tendon becomes gradually softer but does not return to normal levels. Further, elastic properties may be used as biomarkers to evaluate the structural integrity and ultimately the function of tendons, to evaluate the effectiveness of treatments, such as extracorporeal shockwave therapy [35]. Patellar tendinopathy is common among active athletes [36], so sonoelastography may be employed to assist sports medicine clinicians, providing a more effective rehabilitation in athletes with patellar tendinopathy (Fig. 4.2).

4.2.3 Rotator Cuff Tendons

Rotator cuff tears are frequent, affecting about 40% of the population older than 60 years, and are commonly associated with pain and dysfunction [37]. It has been estimated that 20–60% of rotator cuff repairs fail, and the risk for repair failure is higher in patients with larger and more complex tears and with more severe muscle atrophy and fat infiltration. Consequently, preoperative imaging evaluation is essential for a correct surgical planning [38]. Both ultrasound and magnetic resonance imaging are routinely used for evaluating the rotator cuff [39, 40]. In this setting, sonoelastography may provide additional quantitative information about tendon degeneration and

tear chronicity by estimating tissue mechanical properties [41]. Although shear modulus seems not to be clearly associated with any individual variable of supraspinatus tear characteristics (size, tendon retraction) or chronicity (Goutallier grade, occupation ratio), SWE measurements have been shown to be altered in the presence of various tendinopathies [41]. Normal tendons have higher shear modulus than pathologic ones in which stiffness decreases and the presence of signal voids on color elastograms correspond to tendon tears [42–44]. This makes sonoelastography potentially useful when conventional ultrasound is not able to differentiate healthy from pathological tissue, with interesting results also when sonoelastography findings have been compared to magnetic resonance imaging [45–47]. Interestingly, normal supraspinatus tendon SWE velocities (3 m/s ± 0.5) decrease with increasing fat content in the muscle (2.5 m/s ± 0.5; $P = 0.001$) [43]. Further, SE was described to be able to quantify the severity of the fatty infiltration of the supraspinatus, reporting excellent accuracy and inter-observer reliability with a weighted kappa coefficient of 0.81 [45]. Additionally, rotator cuff tendinopathy can be related to muscle stiffness. Indeed, an increased shear modulus at SWE of the upper trapezius muscle has been associated with rotator cuff tendinopathy in a study of volleyball players [48]. These authors suggested that athletes with increased stiffness of the upper trapezius may have a greater risk of developing rotator cuff tendinopathy and, consequently, sonoelastography applied in the upper trapezius might be employed for prevention purposes. Another study found that deltoid muscle softening had a correlation with tendinopathy severity assessed by conventional ultrasound [44]. Moreover, it seems that sonoelastography may offer prognostic utility during the surgical repair planning phase, since supraspinatus fat atrophy, reflected by shear wave modulus, can predict relapsed tears and poor functional outcomes [49]. Then, it was found that quantitative SWE evaluation of the supraspinatus muscle is correlated with the extensibility of the musculotendinous unit on cadaveric shoulders. Thus, sonoelastography could confer a noninvasive method to predict rotator cuff extensibility in the preoperative setting [47]. Last, since late surgical repairs are much more difficult, it might be helpful determining whether a patient is suffering from an acute or chronic rotator cuff tear prior to surgical intervention. Some authors revealed a significant association between elasticity values and the chronicity of symptoms, showing significantly higher elasticity values in torn tendons of patients with chronic shoulder pain.

There was a statistically significant difference in median elasticity according to whether the duration of symptoms was 1 year or less (92 kPa) or longer than 1 year (105 kPa). Therefore, although further studies are warranted, the elasticity and SWE velocity values measured by SWE may be used preoperatively in a comprehensive evaluation of rotator cuff tears that deserve surgical repair [50].

Another common disorder of the rotator cuff that may cause relevant shoulder pain and disability is calcific tendinopathy. It is identified and evaluated with conventional radiography and ultrasound [51, 52]. Imaging guided minimally invasive treatments, such as US-guided percutaneous irrigation of calcific tendinopathy (US-PICT), are effective with about an 80% success rate [53–55]. The evaluation of patients with calcific tendinopathy using SWE allowed defining of a non-dark pattern that was predictor of symptomatic relief after US-PICT. These results suggest the possible role of sonoelastography also in the evaluation and management of rotator cuff calcific tendinopathy [48].

4.2.4 Epicondylar Tendons

Lateral epicondylitis is the most common cause of elbow pain and dysfunction, mainly resulting from continuous microtrauma. It is described as a chronic symptomatic degeneration of the forearm's common extensor tendon attachment at the humeral epicondyle. It is usually associated with repetitive microtrauma from excessive gripping or wrist extension, radial deviation, and/or forearm supination, resulting in multiple microtears of the extensor carpi radialis brevis—the most frequently affected tendon—the pronator and other extensor carpal tendons, leading to a cycle of tendon degeneration and repair [56]. The use of conventional ultrasound to differentiate the pathologic tissue from the healthy one can be challenging because, often, both have the same echogenicity [7, 57]. Previous papers have reported interesting correlations of ES findings with clinical symptom scores and duration, so that the sensitivity of conventional US could be enhanced, when combined with SWE, from 67.1% to 94.3% [30]. Studies using SE and SWE showed a decrease in stiffness patterns on symptomatic tendons, and the

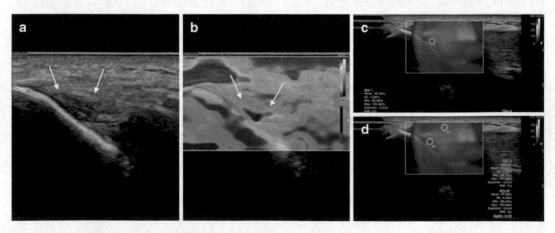

Fig. 4.3 US images of a patient with lateral epicondylitis presenting a small hypoechoic insertional area on B-mode (**a**, arrows) and with yellow and red coloring on the elastogram corresponding to tendon softening (**b**, arrows). Note the stiffness of the pathologic area on SWE calculated as absolute values (**c**) and in ratio with the subcutaneous tissue (**d**)

accuracy of real-time sonoelastography was 94% with clinical examination (Fig. 4.3) [5, 58–62]. In addition, using SE on lateral epicondylitis, more focal lesions, and higher rate of involvement of lateral collateral ligament involvement and peritendinous fascia were reported than using conventional ultrasound alone, highlighting the association of these missed injuries with worse outcomes [58, 63]. Then, studies of epicondylar tendons in cadavers concluded that the combination of sonoelastography and conventional ultrasound provided a better correlation with histology [62, 64]. Elasticity changes on follow-up and rehabilitation treatments should be further evaluated in future research studies, but currently ES is just an additional tool in the detection of lateral epicondylitis (Fig. 4.3).

4.3 Ligaments

Currently, despite the increasing interest in the application of sonoelastography on different musculoskeletal settings and the awareness of the

potential value of this tool, the literature on sonoelastography to image joint ligaments is still relatively scarce. As a general rule, it should be considered that joint positioning plays an important role in ligament sonoelastography imaging because stretched or relaxed ligaments differ substantially. Indeed, normal ligaments in the relaxed state display intermediate SWE velocities (Fig. 4.4), while the velocities increase in the contracted state [65].

4.3.1 Coracohumeral Ligament

Adhesive capsulitis of the shoulder (ACS), also known as frozen shoulder, is characterized by painful gradual loss of both active and passive glenohumeral motion. The underlying cause is not well understood, but it is believed to be characterized by a combination of synovial inflammation and capsular fibrosis. Recent studies believe coracohumeral ligament (CHL) to be critical in the pathology of ACS. Generally, thickening of the CHL and/or the inferior glenohumeral

Fig. 4.4 As an example of the impact of joint positioning on ligament sonoelastography imaging, this case shows the normal B-mode appearance of the ulnar collateral ligament of the elbow in a relaxed state (**a**, arrows) with low SWE velocities (**b**)

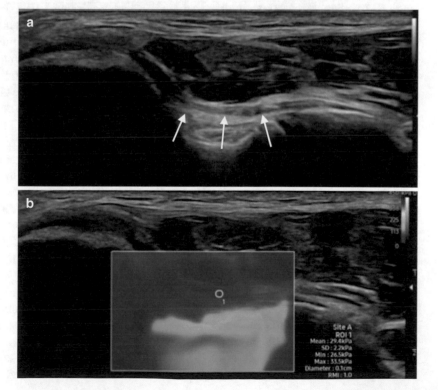

ligament is considered an imaging finding of ACS that can be detected on MRI [66] and ultrasound [67]. However, the identification of subtle changes in these ligaments on conventional ultrasound can be challenging, particularly when the severe restriction of the range of motion affects the execution of the examination. The CHL runs from the lateral base of the coracoid process to the lesser and greater tuberosities of the humerus, forming the roof of the rotator interval. Some authors evaluated the thickness and elasticity of the coracohumeral ligament reporting increased thickness and stiffness of the ligament in patients with ACS [68, 69]. This is coherent with the hypothesis that stiffening of the CHL may play an important role in limiting the range of motion in ACS [70]. ACS can be broken down into 3 stages: stage I (freezing phase), stage II (frozen phase), and stage III (thawing phase). Comparing the SWE measurements of healthy and affected shoulders in the different stages, it was found that the stiffness of the CHL of the affected side was not always greater than that of the healthy shoulder (56–92 kPa). The stiffness of the CHL on the affected side in stage II (median, 166 kPa) and stage III (median, 151 kPa) was higher than that in stage I (median, 89 kPa) ($P < 0.001$), but without any significant differences in the stiffness between stages II and III [71]. Several different treatments are available for frozen shoulder including physiotherapy, steroid injections, hydro-dilatation, manipulation, and arthroscopic capsular release [72]. Notably, in a group of patients successfully treated with ultrasound-guided rotator interval steroid injection, it was observed a reduction in the stiffness of the CHL in both a neutral position and a maximal external rotation [69].

4.3.2 Ankle Ligaments

The lateral ankle ligamentous complex consists of the anterior talofibular ligament (ATFL), calcaneofibular ligament (CFL), and posterior talofibular ligament. The ATFL stabilizes the talus and the CFL stabilizes the subtalar joint. Lateral ankle sprains commonly occur during plantar flexion and inversion with excessive ankle supination, most of these sprains are related to ATFL injury [73]. A recent study defined the normal SWE velocity values for the ATFL and CFL in young male subjects. Based on these results, the SWE mean velocity of the normal ATFL is 2.09 m/s at rest, while that of the normal CFL is 1.99 m/s at rest. Significant differences between the SWE velocities of the two ligaments at rest and stress were found, with increased velocities and tissue stiffness observed with applied stress. Nevertheless, anatomic variations of the ligaments and the interconnection between ligaments and surrounding structures may affect SWE measurements. SWE has shown promising results as a reproducible method to quantify ankle ligament stiffness, but further studies are needed to understand its potential role in pathologic conditions [74]. The main internal stabilizer of the ankle is the medial collateral ligament or deltoid ligament composed of two groups: superficial and deep. The superficial part is composed of the tibio-navicular ligament, the tibio-calcaneal ligament, the anterior part of which is identified as the tibio-spring ligament, and the superficial posterior tibiotalar ligament. The deep part is made of the anterior tibiotalar ligament and the posterior tibiotalar ligament [75]. The integrity of the bundles of the medial ligament complex limits talar abduction, pronation, and external rotation, protecting the syndesmosis and the distal fibula. The deltoid ligament may be injured during traumas occurring in the external rotation of the ankle. The results of an early pilot study suggest that the assessment of the medial ankle ligament complex by SWE is reproducible in healthy subjects. SWE allows a quantitative measurement allowing an assessment of the ligament status in both static and dynamic positions. Thus, it may allow making the initial diagnosis and monitor the effects of rehabilitation by assessing ligament stiffness during follow-up after trauma, but also this application deserves future investigations. Sonoelastography could also help in the preoperative evaluation by selecting the type of graft and adjusting its tension intraoperatively to reproduce as closely as possible the natural ligament stiffness and biomechanical properties described by SWE parameters.

Further works should be conducted to assess the relevance of SWE in the management of medial ankle injuries [76].

4.3.3   Knee Collateral Ligaments

A primary role in stabilizing the knee joint against valgus and varus forces is played by the medial and lateral collateral ligaments. The medial collateral ligament (MCL) can be affected by acute or chronic injuries, and conditions such as inflammation and degeneration. In particular, it is the most common injured ligament in the knee [77]. In athletes, the progression to returning to play after a knee injury is determined by achieving pain-free movement. Nevertheless, the mechanical properties of the recovering ligament are not usually evaluated. A greater awareness of medial collateral ligament elasticity may help orthopedic surgeons. SE represents an easy and reliable tool for measuring the stiffness behavior of the knee collateral ligaments during the rehabilitation phase [78].

The mean stiffness values of the proximal, middle, and distal MCL are about 33 kPa, 35 kPa, and 36 kPa, respectively [79]. The relative stiffness of different portions of the collateral ligaments differs with knee flexion angle because the soft tissues have nonlinear behavior in the general force-displacement curve, therefore it is important to assess strain ratios at various flexion angles. In the superficial and deep medial collateral ligaments, the strain ratio increases with increasing knee flexion, while in the lateral collateral ligament, stiffness shows a tendency to fluctuate. In all three ligaments, strain ratios are lowest at 0° indicating high relative stiffness. Since soft tissues such as ligaments are viscoelastic in nature, their mechanical characteristics may be altered under applied compression, so the use of SWE may avoid this problem. According to a recent study conducted on healthy volunteers, SWE is a feasible, reproducible, and reliable imaging technique useful for the evaluation of the elasticity of the medial collateral ligament. In future studies, data from patients with pathological processes should be collected to recognize deviations from normal [78].

4.3.4   Ulnar Collateral Ligament

The ulnar collateral ligament of the elbow (UCL) is the major stabilizer against valgus stress in overhand [80]. Two articles studied healthy subjects for the characterization of the UCL through sonoelastography [81, 82]. Both concluded that sonoelastography might be useful for evaluating UCL status with the authors recommending further studies to understand the actual role of sonoelastography in detecting UCL injury and in monitoring the healing process during follow-up. According to these studies, the strain ratios for the UCL during gripping and at rest are respectively 17.64 and 3.94, whereas the strain ratios for the FPM during gripping and at rest are respectively 1.72 and 0.35. Sonoelastography measurements of the UCL and flexor pronator muscle (FPM) revealed that the elasticity of the UCL was significantly lower than that of the FPM at rest and during gripping ($P < 0.001$), and both structures showed significantly less elasticity during gripping than at rest ($P < 0.001$). The muscle contraction associated with gripping does not cause a specific change in the elasticity of either the UCL or the FPM at the medial elbow joint, indicating that tissue elasticity is reduced as a whole. This indicates that not only the FPM but also the UCL is tensed during gripping. The proportion of tension for each tissue in the medial elbow joint as a stabilizing contribution against elbow valgus stress is not significantly different between rest and gripping, in fact, no significant difference in the ratio of strain ratios (UCL/FPM) was found between rest and gripping [82]. Further, no significant differences in SWE velocities have been found between the dominant (mean velocity = 5.14 m/s) and non-dominant (mean velocity = 5.24 m/s) arm when examining the UCL [81] (Fig. 4.4).

4.4   Clinical Applications (Table 4.1)

Table 4.1 Summarizes stiffness in most common tendon and ligament pathologies

Clinical scenario	SWE Stiffness values	Source
Achilles tendinopathy/ rupture	Decreased	Aubry et al. [23] and Chen et al. [24]
Surgical repair of Achilles tendon rupture	Increased	Busilacchi et al. [25] and Zhang et al. [26]
Patellar tendinopathy	Equivocal	Dirrichs et al. [30], Rist et al. [31], Ooi et al. [32], Zhang et al. [33], and Porta et al. [34]
Rotator cuff tendinopathy	Decreased especially in chronic lesions with fatty infiltration	Seo et al. [45], Lee et al. [46], Krepkin et al. [47], Bruno et al. [48], Lin et al. [49], and Beeler et al. [50]
Lateral epicondylitis	Decreased	de Zordo et al. [58], Ahn et al. [59], Kang et al. [60], Park et al. [61], Kocyigit et al. [62], and Klauser et al. [63]
Adhesive Capsulitis	Increased CHL stiffness in stages II and III	Zhang et al. [71]
Ulnar collateral ligament injury	Decreased	Gupta et al. [81]

4.5 Conclusion and Future Perspectives

In conclusion, the addition of sonoleatography has proven to provide significant improvement compared with conventional B-mode ultrasound alone in several settings allowing the assessment of mechanical and elastic properties of tendons and ligaments. It might be used to increase the diagnostic performance in the diagnosis and to monitor various conditions during posttreatment follow-up [1]. The evidence supporting the role of sonoelastography in assessing tendons and ligaments is constantly increasing in the literature, but it is still too low, particularly for what concerns ligamentous structures. Further large-

scale studies are needed to ensure validation and clinical application of sonoelastography in tendons and ligaments imaging.

References

1. Taljanovic MS, et al. Shear-wave elastography: basic physics and musculoskeletal applications. Radiographics. 2017;37(3). https://doi.org/10.1148/rg.2017160116.
2. Ooi CC, Malliaras P, Schneider ME, Connell DA. 'Soft, hard, or just right?' Applications and limitations of axial-strain sonoelastography and shear-wave elastography in the assessment of tendon injuries. Skelet Radiol. 2014;43:1. https://doi.org/10.1007/s00256-013-1695-3.
3. Sigrist RMS, Liau J, el Kaffas A, Chammas MC, Willmann JK. Ultrasound elastography: review of techniques and clinical applications. Theranostics. 2017;7(5):1303. https://doi.org/10.7150/thno.18650.
4. Drakonaki EE, Allen GM, Wilson DJ. Ultrasound elastography for musculoskeletal applications. Br J Radiol. 2012;85(1019):1435. https://doi.org/10.1259/bjr/93042867.
5. Klauser AS, Miyamoto H, Bellmann-Weiler R, Feuchtner GM, Wick MC, Jaschke WR. Sonoelastography: musculoskeletal applications. Radiology. 2014;272(3). https://doi.org/10.1148/radiol.14121765.
6. Ryu JA, Jeong WK. Current status of musculoskeletal application of shear wave elastography. Ultrasonography. 2017;36(3):185. https://doi.org/10.14366/usg.16053.
7. Frey H. Realtime elastography. A new ultrasound procedure for the reconstruction of tissue elasticity. Radiologe. 2003;43(10):850.
8. Niitsu M, Michizaki A, Endo A, Takei H, Yanagisawa O. Muscle hardness measurement by using ultrasound elastography: a feasibility study. Acta Radiol. 2011;52(1). https://doi.org/10.1258/ar.2010.100190.
9. Sconfienza LM, et al. Clinical indications for musculoskeletal ultrasound updated in 2017 by European Society of Musculoskeletal Radiology (ESSR) consensus. Eur Radiol. 2018;28(12):5338. https://doi.org/10.1007/s00330-018-5474-3.
10. Götschi T, et al. Region- and degeneration dependent stiffness distribution in intervertebral discs derived by shear wave elastography. J Biomech. 2021;121:110395. https://doi.org/10.1016/j.jbiomech.2021.110395.
11. Gitto S, Messina C, Vitale N, Albano D, Sconfienza LM. Quantitative musculoskeletal ultrasound. Semin Musculoskelet Radiol. 2020;24(4):367. https://doi.org/10.1055/s-0040-1709720.
12. Albano D, et al. Posterior tibial tendon dysfunction: clinical and magnetic resonance imaging findings having histology as reference standard. Eur

J Radiol. 2018;99:55. https://doi.org/10.1016/j.ejrad.2017.12.005.

13. Finnamore E, Waugh C, Solomons L, Ryan M, West C, Scott A. Transverse tendon stiffness is reduced in people with Achilles tendinopathy: a cross-sectional study. PLoS One. 2019;14(2):e0211863. https://doi.org/10.1371/journal.pone.0211863.

14. Gitto S, et al. Superb microvascular imaging (SMI) in the evaluation of musculoskeletal disorders: a systematic review. Radiol Med. 2020;125(5):481. https://doi.org/10.1007/s11547-020-01141-x.

15. Albano D, et al. Magnetic resonance and ultrasound in Achilles tendinopathy: predictive role and response assessment to platelet-rich plasma and adipose-derived stromal vascular fraction injection. Eur J Radiol. 2017;95:130. https://doi.org/10.1016/j.ejrad.2017.08.006.

16. Slane LC, Martin J, DeWall R, Thelen D, Lee K. Quantitative ultrasound mapping of regional variations in shear wave speeds of the aging Achilles tendon. Eur Radiol. 2017;27(2):474. https://doi.org/10.1007/s00330-016-4409-0.

17. Prado-Costa R, Rebelo J, Monteiro-Barroso J, Preto AS. Ultrasound elastography: compression elastography and shear-wave elastography in the assessment of tendon injury. Insights Imaging. 2018;9(5):791. https://doi.org/10.1007/s13244-018-0642-1.

18. Siu WL, Chan CH, Lam CH, Lee CM, Ying M. Sonographic evaluation of the effect of long-term exercise on Achilles tendon stiffness using shear wave elastography. J Sci Med Sport. 2016;19(11):883. https://doi.org/10.1016/j.jsams.2016.02.013.

19. Ruan Z, et al. Elasticity of healthy Achilles tendon decreases with the increase of age as determined by acoustic radiation force impulse imaging. Int J Clin Exp Med. 2015;8(1):1043.

20. Coombes BK, et al. Achilles and patellar tendinopathy display opposite changes in elastic properties: a shear wave elastography study. Scand J Med Sci Sports. 2018;28(3):1201. https://doi.org/10.1111/sms.12986.

21. Chen L, Cheng Y, Liang Z, Zhang L, Deng X. Quantitative shear wave elastography compared to standard ultrasound (qualitative B-mode grayscale sonography and quantitative power Doppler) for evaluation of achillotendinopathy in treatment-naïve individuals: a cross-sectional study. Adv Clin Exp Med. 2022;31:847.

22. Saha D, Prakash M, Sinha A, Singh T, Dogra S, Sharma A. Role of shear-wave elastography in achilles tendon in psoriatic arthritis and its correlation with disease severity score, psoriasis area and severity index. Indian J Radiol Imaging. 2022;32:159.

23. Aubry S, Nueffer JP, Tanter M, Becce F, Vidal C, Michel F. Viscoelasticity in achilles tendonopathy: quantitative assessment by using real-time shear-wave elastography. Radiology. 2015;274(3). https://doi.org/10.1148/radiol.14140434.

24. Chen XM, Cui LG, He P, Shen WW, Qian YJ, Wang JR. Shear wave elastographic characterization of normal and torn Achilles tendons: a pilot study. J Ultrasound Med. 2013;32(3):449. https://doi.org/10.7863/jum.2013.32.3.449.

25. Busilacchi A, et al. Real-time sonoelastography as novel follow-up method in Achilles tendon surgery. Knee Surgery, Sports Traumatology, Arthroscopy. 2016;24(7):2124. https://doi.org/10.1007/s00167-014-3484-5.

26. Zhang LN, et al. Evaluation of elastic stiffness in healing Achilles tendon after surgical repair of a tendon rupture using in vivo ultrasound shear wave elastography. Med Sci Monit. 2016;22:1186. https://doi.org/10.12659/MSM.895674.

27. Breda SJ, van der Vlist A, de Vos RJ, Krestin GP, Oei EHG. The association between patellar tendon stiffness measured with shear-wave elastography and patellar tendinopathy—a case-control study. Eur Radiol. 2020;30(11):5942. https://doi.org/10.1007/s00330-020-06952-0.

28. Lian KJ, Holen LE, Bahr R. Relationship between symptoms of jumper's knee and the ultrasound characteristics of the patellar tendon among high level male volleyball players. Scand J Med Sci Sports. 1996;6(5):291. https://doi.org/10.1111/j.1600-0838.1996.tb00473.x.

29. Cook JL, et al. Patellar tendon ultrasonography in asymptomatic active athletes reveals hypoechoic regions: a study of 320 tendons. Clin J Sport Med. 1998;8(2):73. https://doi.org/10.1097/00042752-199804000-00001.

30. Dirrichs T, Quack V, Gatz M, Tingart M, Kuhl CK, Schrading S. Shear Wave Elastography (SWE) for the evaluation of patients with tendinopathies. Acad Radiol. 2016;23(10):1204. https://doi.org/10.1016/j.acra.2016.05.012.

31. Rist H-J, Mauch M. Quantified TDI elastography of the patellar tendon in athletes. Sportverletz Sportschaden. 2012;26(1):27.

32. Ooi CC, et al. A soft patellar tendon on ultrasound elastography is associated with pain and functional deficit in volleyball players. J Sci Med Sport. 2016;19(5):373. https://doi.org/10.1016/j.jsams.2015.06.003.

33. Zhang ZJ, Ng GYF, Lee WC, Fu SN. Changes in morphological and elastic properties of patellar tendon in athletes with unilateral patellar tendinopathy and their relationships with pain and functional disability. PLoS One. 2014;9(10):e108337. https://doi.org/10.1371/journal.pone.0108337.

34. Porta F, Damjanov N, Galluccio F, Iagnocco A, Matucci-Cerinic M. Ultrasound elastography is a reproducible and feasible tool for the evaluation of the patellar tendon in healthy subjects. Int J Rheum Dis. 2014;17(7):762. https://doi.org/10.1111/1756-185X.12241.

35. Zhang C, Duan L, Liu Q, Zhang W. Correction to: Application of shear wave elastographjy and B-mode ultrasound in patellar tendinopathy after extracorporeal shockwave therapy. J Med Ultrasonics. 2020;47(3):477. https://doi.org/10.1007/s10396-020-01025-7.

36. Peers KHE, Lysens RJJ. Patellar tendinopathy in athletes: current diagnostic and therapeutic recommendations. Sports Med. 2005;35(1):71. https://doi.org/10.2165/00007256-200535010-00006.

37. Roe Y, Bautz-Holter E, Juel NG, Soberg HL. Identification of relevant international classification of functioning, disability and health categories in patients with shoulder pain: a cross-sectional study. J Rehabil Med. 2013;45(7):662. https://doi.org/10.2340/16501977-1159.

38. Choi S, Kim MK, Kim GM, Roh YH, Hwang IK, Kang H. Factors associated with clinical and structural outcomes after arthroscopic rotator cuff repair with a suture bridge technique in medium, large, and massive tears. J Shoulder Elbow Surg. 2014;23(11):1675. https://doi.org/10.1016/j.jse.2014.02.021.

39. Serpi F, Albano D, Rapisarda S, Chianca V, Sconfienza LM, Messina C. Shoulder ultrasound: current concepts and future perspectives. J Ultrasonography. 2021;21(85):e154. https://doi.org/10.15557/JoU.2021.0025.

40. Albano D, et al. Imaging of usual and unusual complication of rotator cuff repair. J Comput Assist Tomogr. 2019;43(3):359. https://doi.org/10.1097/RCT.0000000000000846.

41. Lawrence RL, et al. Ultrasound shear wave elastography and its association with rotator cuff tear characteristics. JSES Int. 2021;5(3):500. https://doi.org/10.1016/j.jseint.2020.11.008.

42. Kocyigit F, Kuyucu E, Kocyigit A, Herek DT, Savkin R, Aslan UB. Investigation of biomechanical characteristics of intact supraspinatus tendons in subacromial impingement syndrome. Am J Phys Med Rehabil. 2016;95(8):588. https://doi.org/10.1097/PHM.0000000000000450.

43. Rosskopf AB, Ehrmann C, Buck FM, Gerber C, Flück M, Pfirrmann CWA. Quantitative shear-wave US elastography of the supraspinatus muscle: reliability of the method and relation to tendon integrity and muscle quality. Radiology. 2016;278(2):465. https://doi.org/10.1148/radiol.2015150908.

44. Hou SW, Merkle AN, Babb JS, McCabe R, Gyftopoulos S, Adler RS. Shear wave ultrasound elastographic evaluation of the rotator cuff tendon. J Ultrasound Med. 2017;36:95. https://doi.org/10.7863/ultra.15.07041.

45. Seo JB, Yoo JS, Ryu JW. The accuracy of sonoelastography in fatty degeneration of the supraspinatus: a comparison of magnetic resonance imaging and conventional ultrasonography. J Ultrasound. 2014;17(4):279. https://doi.org/10.1007/s40477-014-0064-y.

46. Lee SU, Joo SY, Kim SK, Lee SH, Park SR, Jeong C. Real-time sonoelastography in the diagnosis of rotator cuff tendinopathy. J Shoulder Elbow Surg. 2016;25(5):723. https://doi.org/10.1016/j.jse.2015.10.019.

47. Krepkin K, Bruno M, Raya JG, Adler RS, Gyftopoulos S. Quantitative assessment of the supraspinatus tendon on MRI using T2/T2* mapping and shear-wave ultrasound elastography: a pilot study. Skeletal Radiol. 2017;46(2):191. https://doi.org/10.1007/s00256-016-2534-0.

48. Lin YH, Chiou HJ, Wang HK, Lai YC, Chou YH, Chang CY. Management of rotator cuff calcific tendinosis guided by ultrasound elastography. J Chin Med Assoc. 2015;78(10):603. https://doi.org/10.1016/j.jcma.2015.05.006.

49. Beeler S, Ek ETH, Gerber C. A comparative analysis of fatty infiltration and muscle atrophy in patients with chronic rotator cuff tears and suprascapular neuropathy. J Shoulder Elbow Surg. 2013;22(11):1371. https://doi.org/10.1016/j.jse.2013.01.028.

50. Yoo SJ, Lee S, Song Y, Kim CK, Lee BG, Bae J. Elasticity of torn supraspinatus tendons measured by shear wave elastography: a potential surrogate marker of chronicity? Ultrasonography. 2020;39(2):144. https://doi.org/10.14366/usg.19035.

51. Albano D, Coppola A, Gitto S, Rapisarda S, Messina C, Sconfienza LM. Imaging of calcific tendinopathy around the shoulder: usual and unusual presentations and common pitfalls. Radiol Med. 2021;126(4):608. https://doi.org/10.1007/s11547-020-01300-0.

52. Chianca V, et al. Rotator cuff calcific tendinopathy: from diagnosis to treatment. Acta Biomed. 2018;89:186. https://doi.org/10.23750/abm.v89i1-S.7022.

53. Sconfienza LM, et al. Clinical indications for image-guided interventional procedures in the musculoskeletal system: a Delphi-based consensus paper from the European Society of Musculoskeletal Radiology (ESSR)—part VI, foot and ankle. Eur Radiol. 2022;32(2):1488. https://doi.org/10.1007/s00330-021-08125-z.

54. Silvestri E, et al. Interventional therapeutic procedures in the musculoskeletal system: an Italian Survey by the Italian College of Musculoskeletal Radiology. Radiol Med. 2018;123(4):314. https://doi.org/10.1007/s11547-017-0842-7.

55. Tortora S, et al. Ultrasound-guided musculoskeletal interventional procedures around the shoulder. J Ultrason. 2021;21(85):e162. https://doi.org/10.15557/JOU.2021.0026.

56. Ma KL, Wang HQ. Management of lateral epicondylitis: a narrative literature review. Pain Res Manag. 2020;2020:6965381. https://doi.org/10.1155/2020/6965381.

57. Lee HS, et al. Musicians' medicine: musculoskeletal problems in string players. Clin Orthop Surg. 2013;5(3):155. https://doi.org/10.4055/cios.2013.5.3.155.

58. de Zordo T, et al. Real-time sonoelastography of lateral epicondylitis: comparison of findings between patients and healthy volunteers. Am J Roentgenol. 2009;193(1):180. https://doi.org/10.2214/AJR.08.2020.

59. Ahn KS, Kang CH, Hong SJ, Jeong WK. Ultrasound elastography of lateral epicondylosis: clinical fea-

sibility of quantitative elastographic measurements. Am J Roentgenol. 2014;202(5):1094. https://doi.org/10.2214/AJR.13.11003.

60. Park GY, Kwon DR, Park JH. Diagnostic confidence of sonoelastography as adjunct to greyscale ultrasonography in lateral elbow tendinopathy. Chin Med J (Engl). 2014;127(17):3110. https://doi.org/10.3760/cma.j.issn.0366-6999.20140209.

61. Kocyigit F, et al. Association of real-time sonoelastography findings with clinical parameters in lateral epicondylitis. Rheumatol Int. 2016;36(1):91. https://doi.org/10.1007/s00296-015-3356-4.

62. Klauser AS, et al. Extensor tendinopathy of the elbow assessed with sonoelastography: histologic correlation. Eur Radiol. 2017;27(8):3460. https://doi.org/10.1007/s00330-016-4711-x.

63. Clarke AW, Ahmad M, Curtis M, Connell DA. Lateral elbow tendinopathy: correlation of ultrasound findings with pain and functional disability. Am J Sports Med. 2010;38(6):1209. https://doi.org/10.1177/0363546509359066.

64. Klauser AS, et al. Sonoelastography of the common flexor tendon of the elbow with histologic agreement: a cadaveric study. Radiology. 2017;283(2):486. https://doi.org/10.1148/radiol.2016160139.

65. Snoj Ž, Wu CH, Taljanovic MS, Dumić-Čule I, Drakonaki EE, Klauser AS. Ultrasound elastography in musculoskeletal radiology: past, present, and future. Semin Musculoskelet Radiol. 2020;24(2):156. https://doi.org/10.1055/s-0039-3402746.

66. Suh CH, et al. Systematic review and meta-analysis of magnetic resonance imaging features for diagnosis of adhesive capsulitis of the shoulder. Eur Radiol. 2019;29(2):566. https://doi.org/10.1007/s00330-018-5604-y.

67. Wu H, et al. The role of grey-scale ultrasound in the diagnosis of adhesive capsulitis of the shoulder: a systematic review and meta-analysis. Med Ultrason. 2020;22(3):305. https://doi.org/10.11152/mu-2430.

68. Wu CH, Chen WS, Wang TG. Elasticity of the coracohumeral ligament in patients with adhesive capsulitis of the shoulder. Radiology. 2016;278(2):458. https://doi.org/10.1148/radiol.2015150888.

69. McKean D, et al. Elasticity of the coracohumeral ligament in patients with frozen shoulder following rotator interval injection: a case series. J Ultrason. 2020;20(83):e300. https://doi.org/10.15557/JoU.2020.0052.

70. Kanazawa K, et al. Elastic changes of the coracohumeral ligament evaluated with shear wave elastography. Open Orthop J. 2018;12(1):427. https://doi.org/10.2174/1874325001812010427.

71. Zhang J, Zhang L, Guo F, Zhang T. Shear wave elastography of the coracohumeral ligament with frozen shoulder in different stages. J Ultrasound Med. 2022;41(10):2527. https://doi.org/10.1002/jum.15942.

72. Sconfienza LM, Chianca V, Messina C, Albano D, Pozzi G, Bazzocchi A. Upper limb interventions. Radiol Clin North Am. 2019;57(5):1073. https://doi.org/10.1016/j.rcl.2019.05.002.

73. Fong DTP, Hong Y, Chan LK, Yung PSH, Chan KM. A systematic review on ankle injury and ankle sprain in sports. Sports Med. 2007;37(1):73. https://doi.org/10.2165/00007256-200737010-00006.

74. Gimber LH, et al. Ultrasound shear wave elastography of the anterior talofibular and calcaneofibular ligaments in healthy subjects. J Ultrason. 2021;21(85):e86. https://doi.org/10.15557/JoU.2021.0017.

75. Golanó P, et al. Anatomy of the ankle ligaments: a pictorial essay. Knee Surg Sports Traumatol Arthrosc. 2010;18(5):577. https://doi.org/10.1007/s00167-010-1100-x.

76. Rougereau G, et al. A preliminary study to assess the relevance of shear-wave elastography in characterizing biomechanical changes in the deltoid ligament complex in relation to ankle position. Foot Ankle Int. 2022;43(6):840.

77. Bollen S. Epidemiology of knee injuries: diagnosis and triage. Br J Sports Med. 2000;34(3):227. https://doi.org/10.1136/bjsm.34.3.227.

78. Gürün E, Aksakal M, Akdulum İ. Measuring stiffness of normal medial collateral ligament in healthy volunteers via shear wave elastography. Surg Radiol Anat. 2021;43(10):1673. https://doi.org/10.1007/s00276-021-02749-y.

79. Wadugodapitiya S, Sakamoto M, Tanaka M, Sakagami Y, Morise Y, Kobayashi K. Assessment of knee collateral ligament stiffness by strain ultrasound elastography. Biomed Mater Eng. 2022;33(5):337. https://doi.org/10.3233/BME-211282.

80. Morrey BF, An KN. Articular and ligamentous contributions to the stability of the elbow joint. Am J Sports Med. 1983;11(5):315. https://doi.org/10.1177/036354658301100506.

81. Gupta N, et al. Shear-wave elastography of the ulnar collateral ligament of the elbow in healthy volunteers: a pilot study. Skeletal Radiol. 2019;48(8):1241. https://doi.org/10.1007/s00256-019-3162-2.

82. Hattori H, et al. Changes in medial elbow elasticity and joint space gapping during maximal gripping: reliability and validity in evaluation of the medial elbow joint using ultrasound elastography. J Shoulder Elbow Surg. 2020;29(6):e245. https://doi.org/10.1016/j.jse.2019.11.005.

Muscles and Fasciae

5

Ivan Garcia Duitama, Anna Agustí Claramunt, and Pedro Garcia Gonzalez

5.1   Introduction

Nowadays, ultrasound (US) has begun to be one of the most important radiological tools in the assessment of many entities affecting the musculoskeletal system [1]. There is no doubt about the great benefit of using the US for evaluating traumatic muscle injuries and primary muscle pathologies, and following them up to their healing or further degeneration, with the possibility of real-time evaluation, and the advantage of being a radiation-free and inexpensive diagnostic tool [2]. Nevertheless, biomechanical properties of tissues are difficult to assess with B-mode US, even having symptomatic patients [3, 4], and that is why ultrasound elastography may find a role in the path to the diagnosis of, not just traumatic injuries, but also muscle pathologies. In the following chapter, we will point out how elastography may be an added tool for diagnosing muscular entities with ultrasound. To date, there is just one [5] indexed clinical guideline on the Pubmed database regarding the use of ultrasound elastography in the musculoskeletal system, dated 2013,

with just one indication, cerebral spasticity. Further advances since that time have come that we think are worth revising.

Elastography is an ideal added function to the US as a diagnostic test for muscle diseases, as far as it is a noninvasive technique with the ability to quantify the mechanical properties of muscle and can assist clinicians in the diagnosis and evaluation of the progression of diseases and serve as a mean to monitor the effects of treatments [6].

Current literature is trending toward shear wave elastography (SWE) instead of strain elastography (SE) in many fields, and it is expected to be that way in research conditions owing to its capacity to quantify stiffness, which allows comparisons and statistical analysis, as opposed to SE, which offers qualitative information. Nevertheless, since elastography isn't in many clinical guidelines, not all the scanners in daily practice offer that functionality, particularly older models; in the field of musculoskeletal imaging some devices offer SE, some SWE, or even, they may not be equipped with elastography at all. We think it is important to stress that it is not always mandatory to measure the stiffness of tissues, sometimes the color-coded elastogram may give us the added information needed to diagnose or follow a particular case, and for that purpose, we can use the contralateral side of the patient as a control, an intrinsic advantage in the assessment of the musculoskeletal system.

I. G. Duitama (✉) · A. A. Claramunt
Department of Radiodiagnostic, Hospital del Mar, Barcelona, Spain
e-mail: igarciaduitama@psmar.cat

P. G. Gonzalez
Department of Radiology, Clínica Molinón, Gijón, Asturias, Spain

© The Author(s), under exclusive license to Springer Nature Switzerland AG 2023
S. Marsico, A. Solano (eds.), *Elastography of the Musculoskeletal System*,
https://doi.org/10.1007/978-3-031-31054-6_5

5.1.1 Peculiarities of Muscle and Fascia Affecting Elastography and Practical Recommendations

Many features of muscle and fasciae significantly influence the elastographic evaluation of such structures; they can be related to mechanical, histologic, anatomic, pathologic, variations between individuals, and the sampling technique [7].

Muscle fibers, collagen, and myofibrils are arranged in longitudinal units that confer significant anisotropic properties to the muscles. Shear waves propagate easier when examined in the parallel than in the perpendicular plane, with significantly higher stiffness values in the short axis than in the longitudinal axis (Fig. 5.1). Also,

measuring muscular modulus in the transverse plane, relative to the muscle's longitudinal axis, can comprise inter and intra-observer reproducibility [8]. Furthermore, muscle inner arrangement of fibers is varied, from parallel, fan-shaped, circular, pennate (feather-like), multipenneate to fusiform [9], a factor that introduces a technical difficulty at the time of standardizing the examination technique. Because of that fact, if elastography is used to compare muscle modulus to a previous value in the same patient, or a published standard, measurements need to be done by scanning the muscle in the same axis used in the control exam [10].

Muscles are dynamic units that change their stiffness depending on their state at the time of sampling, increasing during contraction and

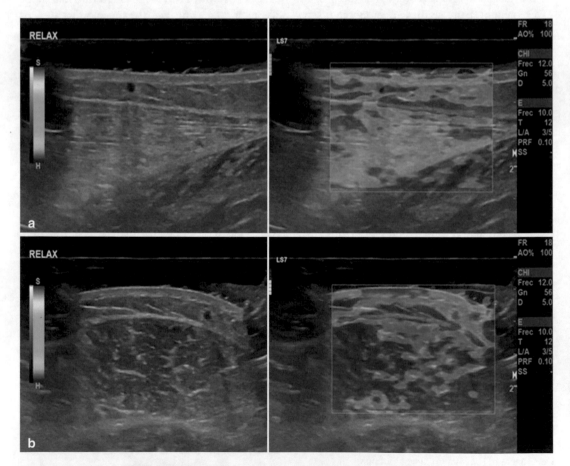

Fig. 5.1 Elastogram of normal muscle in the transverse (**a**) and longitudinal (**b**) planes of the medial gastrocnemius in a relaxed position. B-mode is shown on the left side and the corresponding elastogram is on the right. Note there is an apparent increase in muscle stiffness in the transverse plane

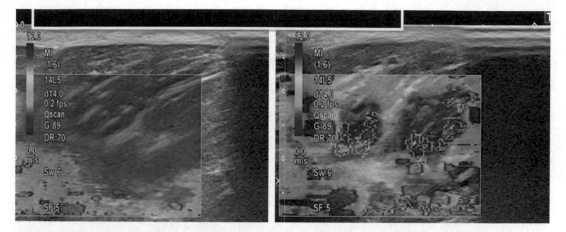

Fig. 5.2 Elastographic variation with muscle contraction. Elastograms of the biceps femoris muscle in a plane paralleling muscle fibers. Note the increased stiffness detection during muscle contraction (right), compared to the resting state (left). The elastogram colors move upward in the stiffness scales, indicating increased stiffness

maximal extension, and decreasing when in a relaxed state [11, 12] (Fig. 5.2). According to the results of Wang et al. [13], the shear modulus of the vastus intermedius does not change significantly in the relaxed state between elderly and young healthy individuals, nevertheless, in younger individuals, the stiffness is greater than in the elderly during contraction. Although it makes sense biologically, such results can't apply to all muscles [14]. Interestingly, SWE can be used as a technique for measuring slow muscle contractions, as it can generate elastograms at a speed of 1 Hz [6].

Good reproducibility of results can be obtained with SWE [8, 12, 15], but it is mandatory to systematically evaluate each muscle following the same patient and probe positioning if their elastographic modulus values or elastograms are intended to be compared to an index value or used in the follow-up of a given individual.

Finally, It is important to note that in SWE, the stiffness can be expressed by different manufacturers as Young's modulus (kPa), shear modulus (kPa), or shear wave velocity (m·s^{-1}), all of them correlated positively [7]. Contrary to the classic recommendation of applying a generous amount of gel to perform US elastography [7], according to Abdulrahman et al. results [16], in the evaluation of muscles, the best reliability is yielded by using the shear wave velocity as the unit of measurement, applying minimal probe load instead of using a standoff gel, and in depths less than 4 cm.

5.1.2 Elastography of the Normal Muscle and Fascia

In normal conditions, muscle has a heterogenous, although organized US B mode appearance, produced by the many tissue interfaces between the muscle fibers and fascicles, and the interstitial structures like perimysium and fasciae. Those interstitial structures are essential for muscle function because they transmit the force generated in muscle fibers to tendons and bones. Also, nerves and vessels traverse muscles and fascial and interfascial plains, providing more image heterogeneity. Such tissue heterogeneity of the normal muscle is also seen in the US strain elastograms, with muscle fibers accounting for the majority of the image, corresponding to low stiffness, and interspersed fibrofatty interstitium and fasciae between the muscle fibers and bellies, of higher stiffness [17, 18]. Nevertheless, the shear wave elastogram of the normal muscle is more homogenous (Fig. 5.3).

The term "fascia" is broad and differentiates fascia itself from the fascial system [19]. For this chapter, we will call fascia only the deep fascia, specially epimysium, the interstitial membrane encasing individual muscles, and aponeurosis, a

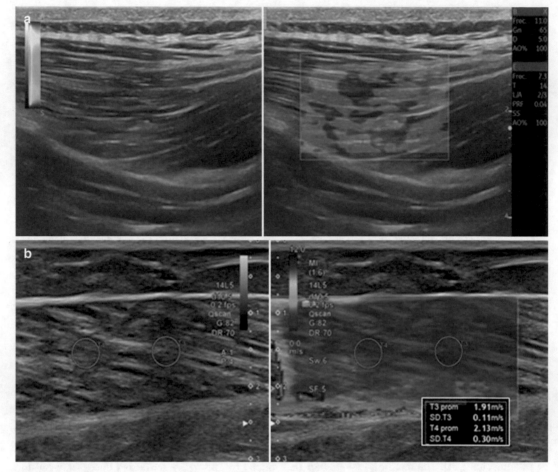

Fig. 5.3 Strain elastogram (image in the right square in **a** and both images in **b**) of healthy muscle and corresponding B mode ultrasound imaging (image in the left square in **a**). Quadratus lumborum muscle in the longitudinal plane with the patient in the prone and relaxed position. With this equipment, the elastographic pattern appears heterogeneous

fascial expansion to attach muscles that require wide attachment to bones or other muscles. Other components in the fascial system will be referred to as interstitium, encasing endomysium, epimysium, perimysium, and interfascial planes. Although joint capsules, tendons, and ligaments, belong to the fascial system according to the current Fascia Research Society glossary [20], they will not be discussed in this chapter.

Finally, it is fair to acknowledge the effort made by many investigations to establish normality values of shear wave elastography corresponding to different muscles along the human anatomy, with varied values corresponding to different muscles, and patient and probe positioning, which soon could provide a reference for comparison in clinical practice or new research projects [7] (Table 5.1).

Table 5.1 Elastography of different muscles and exploration technique applied

	Shear wave elastography measurement	Exploration technique	Source
Medial gastrocnemius	27. 6 ± 7.3 kPa (YM)	Prone position, 30° of passive ankle plantar flexion, transverse plane.	Akagi [21]
Lateral gastrocnemius	33.5 ± 6.3 kPa (YM)	Prone position, 30° of passive ankle plantar flexion, transverse plane.	Akagi [21]
Lateral gastrocnemius	Men: 3.134 ± 1.06 kPa; women: 2.499 ± 1.03 kPa (SWM)	Prone position, 20° of passive ankle plantar flexion, longitudinal plane.	Akagi [22]
Soleus	Men: 3.561 ± 0.8 kPa; women: 2.979 ± 0.8 kPa (SWM)	Prone position, 20° of passive ankle plantar flexion, longitudinal plane.	Akagi [22]
Rectus femoris	Men: 3.439 ± 0.66 kPa; women: 3.182 ± 0.57 kPa (SWM)	Supine position, hips and knees extended, ankles on a cushion, longitudinal.	Akagi [22]
Rectus femoris	8.6 kPa (mean SWM)	Supine. Oriented in the direction of contraction of the muscle fibers, during maximal voluntary contraction.	Bouillard [23]
Rectus femoris	1.8 m/s (SWS)	Supine. Relaxed state. Longitudinal paralleling muscle fibers, from the lateral side of the muscle.	Alfuraih, 2017 [24]
Vastus lateralis	17.45 kPa (mean SWM)	Prone. Longitudinal, during maximal voluntary contraction.	Bouillard [23]
Vastus lateralis	Rest: 1.7 m/s; passive stretch: 1.79 m/s (median SWS)	Supine. Longitudinal. Rest: Knee extended. Passive stretch: Knee flexed 45°.	Paramalingam [25]
Vastus medialis	11.9 kPa (mean SWM)	Longitudinal, during maximal voluntary contraction	Bouillard [23]
Supraspinatus	2.6 ± 0.3	Transverse plane, patient sitting with arm resting on the ipsilateral thigh.	Rosskopf [26]
Deltoid	Rest: 2.3 m/s; passive stretch 2.8 m/s (median SWS)	Longitudinal. Rest: Elbow flexed, resting on a pillow. Passive stretch: Arm hanging freely, elbow extended.	Paramalingam [25]

YM Young's modulus, *SWM* shear wave modulus, *SWS* shear wave speed. All of these values were obtained from healthy young adults

5.2 Clinical Applications

A summary of the findings in different clinical conditions can be found in Table 5.2.

5.2.1 Primary and Secondary Muscle Disorders

In this section, we will speak about a heterogeneous group of diseases that share their affinity for muscle involvement, giving rise to a varied spectrum of clinical conditions in which knowing the biomechanics of the muscle can help the clinician to establish the current state of the disease and guide the therapeutic strategy.

Table 5.2 Summary of elastographic findings in different conditions

Clinical scenario	Stiffness behavior
Idiopathic inflammatory myositis	Decreased
Cerebral palsy	Increased
Duchenne dystrophy	Increased
Acute muscle tear	Decreased
Subacute muscle tear	Increased
Chronic muscle scar	Normal or increased
Painful tense muscle	Variable—increased
Sarcopenia	Decreased in early stages—increased in late stages
Plantar fasciitis	Decreased
Compartment syndrome	Increased x 2–9 times the contralateral side

5.2.1.1 Inflammatory Myositis

Idiopathic inflammatory myopathies (IIM) are a rare group of acquired skeletal muscle diseases, unified by immune-mediated muscle damage, that results in muscle fiber loss and weakness, including a broad spectrum of diseases such as inclusion body myositis, polymyositis, dermatomyositis, and even thyroid disorders. However, all of them share clinical presentations in the form of subacute or chronic muscle weakness courses and a biopsy with the presence of inflammatory infiltrates or disorders that suggest an immune-mediated cause. Most of them are pathologies that should be diagnosed early because they could receive curative treatment. These diseases are diagnosed from a combination of clinical presentation, laboratory tests, and biopsy [27, 28]. The main diagnostic target would be to be able to monitor the inflammatory load. A good correlation was found between elastography and specific muscle biomarkers like the levels of creatine kinase (CK) and lactate dehydrogenase (LDH) [29]. Despite the subtypes of IIM, with heterogeneous clinical and muscular involvement, they share the same pattern of findings, consisting of inflammation/edema, followed by fatty infiltration and eventually muscle atrophy. Some studies focus on the deltoid and vastus lateralis muscles, because of their common involvement in IIM, showing lower values of shear wave speed in these patients, compared to healthy controls [25]. Song et al. [30] found a significant correlation between semi-quantitative US strain elastography rates and pathological scores in biopsy samples in patients with IIM. In that study they could not find a significant correlation with qualitative US and magnetic resonance imaging (MRI) analysis, stressing the added value of elastography in the evaluation of these patients, especially in the early stages of the disease. Finally, a significant advantage of elastography is that it allows monitoring the evolution of the disease in a simple and noninvasive way.

5.2.1.2 Duchenne Dystrophy

Inherited myopathies and muscular dystrophies encase a varied group of diseases with a genetic origin, that present with weakness, motor delay, and respiratory and bulbar dysfunction. Duchenne dystrophy is the most common among them, with a prevalence of 1/3300 males [31]. In Duchenne dystrophy, there is an involvement of the dystrophin gene that makes muscle contraction impossible and clinically manifests itself with proximal weakness, already evident at a very early age, about 5 years, leading to the impossibility of independent ambulation over 13 years without treatment, with early cardiorespiratory involvement that implies high morbidity and mortality in adolescent age. The affected musculature presents an excessive deposit of fibroadipose tissue, with loss of muscle mass and its function, showing atrophy and diffuse increase in echogenicity in B mode ultrasound, as well as an increase in stiffness in the elastographic evaluation. There is a characteristic pattern of involvement: predominant in gluteus maximus and quadriceps muscles with relative sparing of the gracilis, sartorius, and semimembranosus muscles and, in the lower leg, predominant in the superficial posterolateral muscles more than the deep posterior and anterior leg muscles. SWE measurements are generally increased compared to age-matched controls, especially the gluteus maximus (*mean 27 kPa versus 21.9 kPa*), and tibialis anterior muscles (*mean 96.8 kPa versus 23.1 kPa*) [32]. Furthermore, a study analyzed changes in SWE values in patients with DMD over 12 months, and elastography proved to be a good candidate for a monitoring tool [33].

5.2.1.3 Cerebral Palsy

Cerebral palsy (CP) is a nonprogressive (though not unchanging) disorder of movement and posture pathology associated with an impairment of the developing fetal or infant brain (up to 2 years old). It represents the first cause of disability in childhood. It has a prevalence of 1.5–2.5 per 1000 live births and is estimated to affect around 17 million people worldwide. Although the symptoms can be very diverse depending on the brain involvement (motor deficit, epilepsy, behavioral changes, etc.), some of the most frequent complications are musculoskeletal deformations and hypertonia (spasticity, dystonia, and

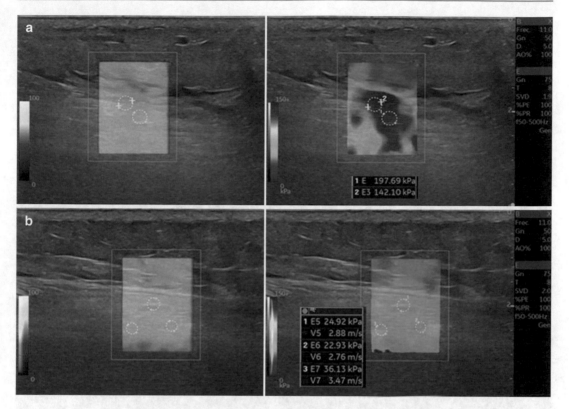

Fig. 5.4 Shear wave elastography in an adult patient affected by cerebral palsy. In B mode the medial and lateral gastrocnemius muscles appear equally hyperechogenic, as seen on the background of the elastograms. The medial gastrocnemius (**a**) showed a shear modulus between 142 and 197 kPa, whereas the lateral gastrocnemius (**b**) showed a shear modulus between 24 and 36 kPa. This reflects an asymmetric involvement of these muscles, probably with a larger amount of fibrosis in the medial gastrocnemius. Note that in healthy individuals, the stiffness is greater in the lateral gastrocnemius

stiffness) [34, 35]. CP is one of the most common disorders associated with secondary muscle changes. It has been shown that patients with CP have greater shear modulus (rigidity) and also that there is more variability in stiffness than in patients without CP [36]. It has also been demonstrated significantly different shear wave speeds between the less and more affected sides [37], and that muscle stiffness assessed using elastography is related to clinical presentations according to the MAS score (modified Ashworth scale) [38], which measures clinically the resistance during passive soft tissue stretching and it is used as a simple measure of spasticity. Given that the most frequent subtype of cerebral palsy is that associated with spasticity, the target in these cases is to be able to guide the rehabilitation techniques on which the treatment is based, and also

to monitor the botulin toxin A (BoNT-A) treatment. Clear associations between post-BoNT-A changes in elastography measurements and clinical scale scores for spasticity have been proved [39]. Also, elastography can be useful to plan the best interval between doses as it has been used to quantify the duration of treatment effect, resulting in <3 months post injection [40] (Fig. 5.4).

5.2.2   Traumatic Muscle Injury

Muscle injuries have three pathophysiologic phases: destructive, reparative, and remodeling. The destructive phase takes place at the time of the injury, depending on the severity of the lesion it will produce or not a hematoma in situ and a separation gap between muscle fibers/interstitium stumps. The reparative phase occurs around the second day after an injury and produces a scar, revascularization, and regeneration of myofibrils at the site of the lesion. The remodeling phase occurs later when the scar tissue reorganizes and the regenerated myofibrils maturate, leading to the recovery of muscle function. In US elastography, the destructive phase will show the injured tissue as a focal decrease in muscle stiffness, corresponding to the hematoma, and overdistended or torn myofibrils. Small tears may be difficult to detect with B mode US, however, the elastogram can show the softened area, confirming the diagnosis. In the reparative phase, the elastography will depict the scar tissue as an area of increased stiffness that can extend beyond the injury seen in B mode US [41–43]. Furthermore, it has been suggested as a good prognostic sign, the presence of decreased stiffness muscle adjacent to the scar tissue seen on B mode US ("elastic ribbed appearance"), as it is less prone to

re-injury and behaves biomechanically better during contraction [41, 42] (Figs. 5.5 and 5.6).

Fascial tissues, including the rest of the interstitium, have viscoelastic and inhomogeneous properties that affect their biomechanics even more than myofibrils. The loose component in the interstitium works as a sliding system and accounts for its viscous properties. Also, in normal conditions, the fascial tissues change their elastographic behavior depending on the position of the joints related to their insertions. For instance, the gastrocnemius's fasciae appear soft in a relaxed state and progressively and significantly increase their stiffness according to different degrees of ankle dorsiflexion [44], a factor that needs to be taken into account when performing the study (Fig. 5.7).

After a fascia injury, the elastographic changes occur following the same phases described above in the case of muscle injury. Well, in the chronic phase the fibrotic tissue and the altered loose

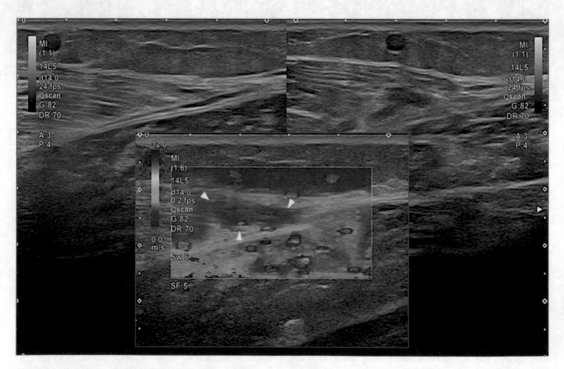

Fig. 5.5 This is a patient with insidious onset pain after prolonged exercise. The ultrasound (on the left) is practically normal, however, the elastography (below) shows focal softening. During contraction (on the right) a

hypoechoic zone (dashed line) is observed that corresponds to a tear and coincides with the softening depicted in the shear wave elastogram

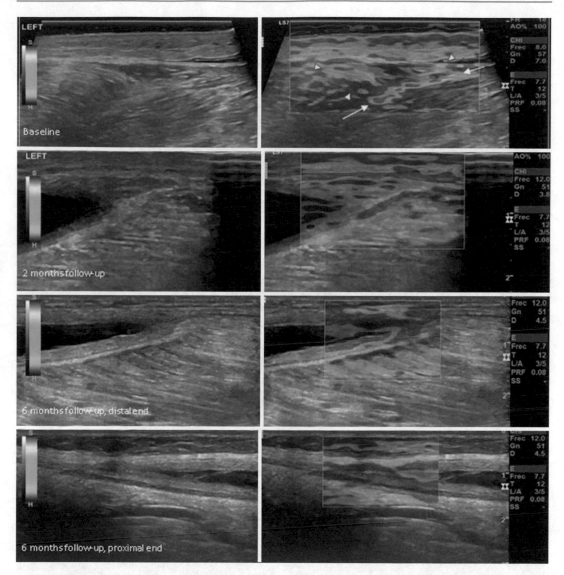

Fig. 5.6 Evolution of a sports injury of medial gastrocnemius, "tennis leg." US B-mode and corresponding strain elastogram images in the longitudinal plane of the distal medial gastrocnemius aponeurosis. The first US demonstrated a distal myoaponeurotic tear with focal softening of the injured tissues. Note the green area corresponding to the hematoma and muscle stumps (arrowheads), and the "red" softened fascia (arrows). In the 2 months follow-up study, a massive hematoma extending proximally through the myofascial junction and deep venous thrombosis (not shown) were detected. The elastogram showed a softened myoaponeurotic junction, indicating immature scaring. At 6 months follow-up the patient still has mild symptoms, the hematoma significantly diminished but the scarring process is incomplete and heterogeneous. At the distal end, the scar has areas of softening and the underlying muscle is hard. At the proximal end, the fascial scar stiffness is comparable to the normal fascia, and the underlying muscle has a normal pattern

interstitial component can become stiffer than normal tissue, losing sliding properties and sometimes affecting the muscle function, a phenomenon that patients may refer to as "tightness"[45] (Fig. 5.8).

Nerve endings run through the interstitium. The neuromuscular system is based on sensory information that allows measuring the length and speed of muscle fibers constantly, thus maintaining tension and being sensitive to stretching in all

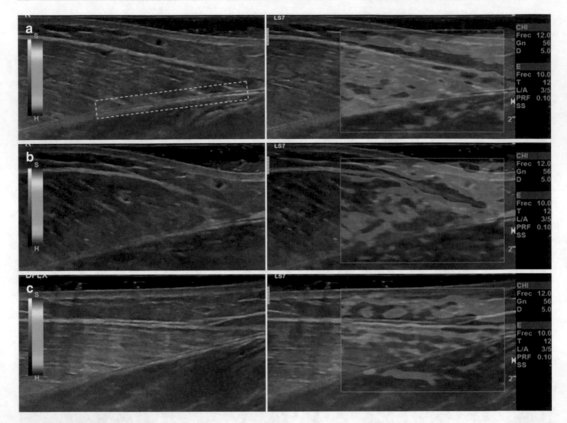

Fig. 5.7 Elastographic changes in gastrocnemius fascia according to the position of the joints. (**a**) Relaxed state. (**b**) Active contraction, (**c**) ankle dorsiflexion. B-mode on the left and strain elastogram on the right. The dashed box encases the deep fascia of the medial gastrocnemius. In the relaxed position, the fascia appears with an intermediate softness (green), and in active contraction and ankle dorsiflexion, the stiffness increases both in the muscle and in the fascia (blue)

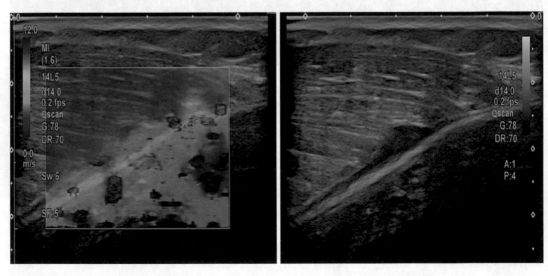

Fig. 5.8 This is a patient with a previous tennis leg injury who undergoes a follow-up ultrasound. B-mode US continues to show a nonspecific hypoechoic area. Shear wave elastography demonstrates stiff scar tissue in the myoaponeurotic junction, indicating a mature scar. Nevertheless, there is also increased stiffness in the soleus muscle, as opposed to the good prognostic "elastic ribbed appearance" sign, indicating in this case, incomplete restoration of the aponeurosis properties

phases of contraction and relaxation. Hyperexcitability of the motor neuron can lead to spastic hypertonia when muscle responsiveness is impaired [6]. Also, the modification in the sliding properties of the interstitium after a muscle injury can lead to abnormal movement of the nociceptors within it during muscle function, and misinterpret such mechanical dysfunction as pain [45].

In terms of return-to-play time, the goal is to achieve muscle function restoration before restarting the sports practice. Based on MRI and medical records, previous studies showed return-to-play times between a few days and 7 weeks for calf injuries [46, 47], probably reflecting heterogeneity in the inclusion of pure muscular and myotendinous junction injuries, the latter known to have a longer repairing time [48]. Yoshida et al. [49] found that musculotendinous junction injuries in the calf tend to restore their normal stiffness between 8 and 12 weeks, longer than previous reports. A possible application for this finding is to follow up with elastography on the healing process of the myotendinous junction's injury to guide the optimal return-to-play time, avoiding potential re-injury.

Blunt trauma has been studied in animals with SWE demonstrating a transient increase in muscle stiffness after the traumatic injury, that correlated with increased collagen fibers (fibrosis). Fibrosis was found to be higher in the group without treatment than in the treatment group. Thus, elastography could be used to demonstrate the tissue alterations after blunt trauma, follow the recovery phase, and monitor the response to therapies [50].

Literature is limited in using SWE in patients with delayed onset muscle soreness (DOMS), a type of transient muscle injury induced by extenuating exercise. So far, US elastography does not appear to have a practical application in this field. It has been found a transient increase in muscle stiffness after vigorous exercise under controlled conditions [51–53], nevertheless, Agten et al. did not find a correlation between the observed increase in stiffness suffered by the affected muscles and clinical symptoms nor quantitative MRI parameters, which by counterpart, had significant correlation with pain [53].

5.2.3 Painful Muscle Disorders

Regional myofascial pain is a clinical syndrome characterized by the development of pain related to trigger points [54]. Although its exact etiology is not fully known, it appears to be related to a protracted spontaneous contraction of a selected muscle band (taut band), that leads to ischemia in the affected muscle, which in turn activates nociceptors and produces pain, in a vicious cycle. The main goal of the management is to stop that cycle. Previous publications showed how the US can demonstrate these trigger points, as hypoechoic rounded areas with altered echotexture [55], and nowadays with the added tool of SWE, we can also measure their stiffness. As shown by Ertekin et al. [56] SWE is a suitable test to detect latent trigger points, clinically silent points that may convert into active and symptomatic [57], and to monitor the effects of physical therapy, referred to by them as the most effective treatment option, demonstrating a significant decline in muscle stiffness, accompanying a clinical improvement, after 4 weeks of treatment. Nevertheless, literature is limited in this field and the study by Valera-Calero et al. [58] did not find a significant correlation between muscle stiffness measured by SWE and clinical severity markers, although they demonstrated increased stiffness in the trigger points and also in the rest of the affected muscle. That said, more research is needed to clarify the actual utility of demonstrating the increased stiffness in trigger points and muscles of patients suffering from this syndrome.

Additionally, elastography can be used to demonstrate muscle tension, a painful syndrome that is readily common in daily practice. Some studies have investigated this topic, but so far, the results have not been homogeneous demonstrating increased or decreased stiffness in the painful areas, although there were differences in the methodological approach to measurements. The relationship seems more constant in the case of neck and back pain, in which increased stiffness can be readily observed with SE [59] (Fig. 5.9). This finding could be used in the future to guide therapies and follow-up their effects.

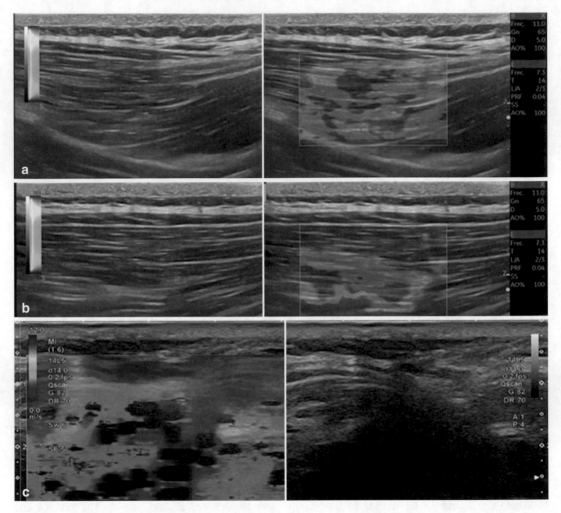

Fig. 5.9 Examples of painful muscle tension. (a and b) belongs to a patient with acute lumbar back pain. (a) is longitudinal imaging of the left quadratus lumborum muscle, with B-mode and corresponding strain elastogram. The elastographic pattern of the muscle is normal. (b) shows the symptomatic right quadratus lumborum, with diffusely increased stiffness. (c) Another patient with left cervical pain, in which the shear wave elastogram in the transverse plane, shows diffusely increased stiffness in the left multifidus muscle

5.2.4 Acute Compartment Syndrome

Acute compartment syndrome (ACS) is an orthopedic emergency caused by increased interstitial pressure, the intracompartmental pressure (ICP), in a closed osteofascial compartment, usually affecting the limbs. It can be derived from many causes, like fractures or compression injuries, that lead to hypoxia, with potentially serious consequences if untreated, like muscular necrosis, limb dysfunction, amputation, and death [60].

The diagnosis is difficult, usually clinical and invasive methods, like Whitesides needle intra-compartmental manometry [61]. SWE is a promising tool to assess the ICP as found by Zhang et al. [62], they manage to demonstrate a statistically significant increase in muscular stiffness in patients with suspected ACS from many causes. In their study, the group treated with fasciotomy showed a several times increase in Young's modulus of the affected compartment, compared to the unaffected limb, ranging from 2 to 9.74. At the time of writing this chapter, there are ongoing studies in this field with unpublished results, that we hope to support the described findings, and enhance the potential role of SWE in such cases, providing a clinical guide to diagnosis and treatment.

5.2.5 Plantar Fasciitis

This is a self-limiting but life-altering condition in which a painful sensation is felt when pressing on the heel, exacerbated by periods of non-loading. It is the most common cause of nontraumatic heel pain and develops after degeneration of the plantar fascia at its calcaneal enthesis due to multifactorial causes. The diagnosis can usually be sufficed by clinical history and physical examination, nevertheless, the US can confirm the diagnosis and guide minimally invasive treatments [63–65]. As described in a recent meta-analysis by Wu et al. [66], the plantar fascia is significantly less stiff in patients with plantar fasciitis than in asymptomatic individuals (Fig. 5.10). They found this feature can be demonstrated both with SE and SWE, although further investigations are needed to evaluate the impact of this finding in the diagnosis and treatment of patients with plantar fasciitis.

5.2.6 Sarcopenia

Sarcopenia is defined by the European Working Group on Sarcopenia in Older People (EWGSOP), as *a syndrome characterised by progressive and generalized loss of skeletal muscle mass and strength, with a risk of adverse outcomes as physical disability, falls, fractures, poor quality of life and death* [67, 68]. Its prevalence is increasing, reaching up to 50% of the population older than 80 years [69]. Changes in muscle parameters can start as early as 25, but it is beyond 60, when muscle quantity, quality, and strength begin to decline considerably. Its diagnosis relies on the determination of low muscle strength and, low muscle quantity or quality, and is considered severe when low physical performance is detected [69]. From the imaging side, diagnosis of low muscle quantity may be established by dual X-ray absorptiometry (DXA), CT, MRI, and US [70]. DXA is probably the most accepted imaging test for determining sarcopenia, owing to the validated cut-off values that make it useful in clinical practice. Limitations of DXA include poor evaluation of muscle quality in terms of muscle steatosis, and the fact that may be biased in patients with extracellular water accumulation as those

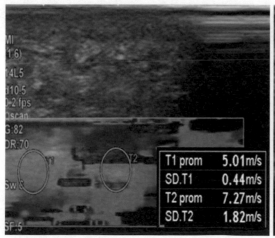
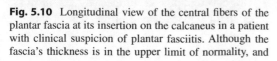
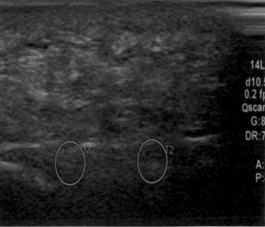

Fig. 5.10 Longitudinal view of the central fibers of the plantar fascia at its insertion on the calcaneus in a patient with clinical suspicion of plantar fasciitis. Although the fascia's thickness is in the upper limit of normality, and consequently of doubtful imaging diagnosis, the shear wave elastography showed significantly reduced stiffness at the insertional portion compared to the distal portion, confirming the diagnosis of plantar fasciitis

with heart, kidney, and liver failure because DXA cannot differentiate water from lean mass, the key parameter that estimates the amount of non-fatty/non-bony tissues the body [71, 72]. CT is becoming a recurrent tool in many studies to measure muscle quantity, in terms of cross-sectional area, and quality, in terms of muscle density, recognizing that abnormal muscle decrease in area and density. It has the disadvantages of using radiation, being unavailable in some clinical settings, and being unable to work by the patient's bedside. MRI is a promising tool for the determination of sarcopenia because of the possibility of evaluating muscle quantity and quality with semi-quantitative and quantitative sequences, without the need for radiation exposure. Though, its use is so far limited to research conditions and shares the limitations of unavailability and inability of bedside exploration, has long acquisition times, and there is a lack of cut-off values and standardized protocols [70]. Ultrasound assessment can detect reduced quantity, and quality in the form of volume loss, increased echogenicity reflecting fat infiltration, and changes in pennation angle and fascicle length. US SWE has been proposed as an added tool to measure muscle quality, considering that muscle stiffness reduces while different grades of fatty infiltration occur until it gets completely infiltrated and atrophied, when the stiffness increases, as shown in the case of rotator cuff tendon rupture and associated muscle degeneration [26]. Although the relation between muscle stiffness and aging is still not completely clear, studies show a higher stiffness in the older population [14]. Results show great variability probably due to different techniques, different muscular groups studied, differences in activity level, and different ages in the target population. Sarcopenia determination with ultrasound and SWE is promising because it could overpass disadvantages of CT and MRI, like radiation, high cost, and long acquisition time, but so far shares with them a lack of validated cut-off values, which limits its use in clinical practice [70, 73].

5.3   Limitations

As with any other diagnostic test, elastography has some specific limitations for the evaluation of muscles that should be known in advance, as well as the technical recommendations to avoid them as much as possible [74].

- SWE measurements may vary from one vendor to another. Although the found variation is minimal, it is unclear if it could be clinically relevant or not [24, 75]. In case of following-up patients or research conditions, use the same equipment to avoid such variability.
- Skin overpressure may increase the measured stiffness in muscle. When scanning, apply as minimal pressure as possible [76].
- Variability in measurements due to the scanning angle. Most reproducibility is yielded by measuring stiffness in the longitudinal plane [24] and < 30° relative to muscle fibers orientation [77].
- Vigorous exercise transiently increases muscle stiffness. Then, if the patients to be tested have exercised, wait at least 48 h after strenuous physical activity, when muscle stiffness returns to baseline [78].
- Small ROI increases variance in SWE results. The use of a medium-sized ROI (defined as one with an area of 75 mm^2) was found to produce better intra-observer agreement [24].
- Soft tissues over convex bony surfaces may have artificially altered stiffness. To avoid such artifact reorientation of the probe is advised, selecting a scanning area where the bony surface isn't convex or measuring far from the artifact band ("reflective corridor") [79].
- As occurs with B-mode US, the deeper the tissues evaluated, the more US/Shear Waves attenuation (5). Scanning tissues obtain the best results at <4 cm deep [16]. In fact, in patients with thick subcutaneous tissue, elastography may not reach the muscle (Fig. 5.11).
- US elastography is limited by its intrinsic operator dependency and the risk of lacking

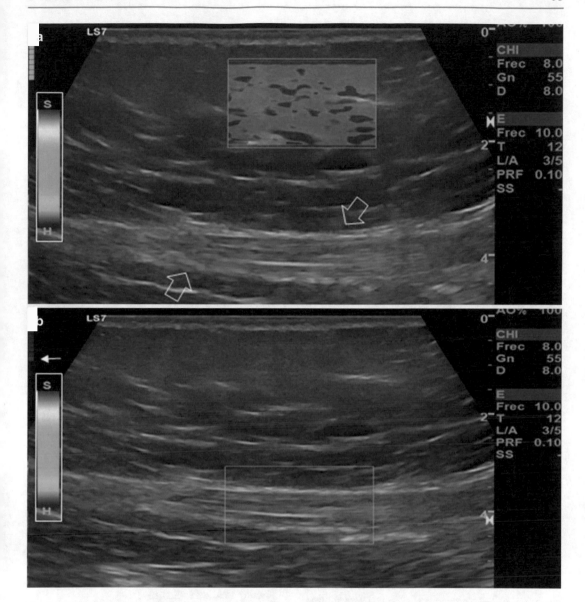

Fig. 5.11 Limitation of elastography due to thick subcutaneous tissue. US study of the abdominal wall in an obese patient. (**a**) Strain elastography of the subcutaneous fat. (**b**) Strain elastography of the rectus abdominis muscle (void arrow), about 3.5 cm from the skin surface. Note the quality sensor indicates poor sampling (arrowhead) and the elastogram is not presented (empty box)

reproducibility [18]. Do your best to be consistent in performing the test, do 3–5 measurements, and use the mean value. Practice makes perfect: better intra-operator agreement has been found in the case of experienced operators [8].

- US elastography is affected by the "eggshell effect," in which harder tissues surrounding a

ROI limit the penetration of the compression wave [79]. As far as technically possible, avoid scanning around bony surfaces.

- Movement of the patient or the probe during the test can produce unreliable results. Try scanning in a stable position and do 3–5 measurements to detect possible motion artifacts [79].

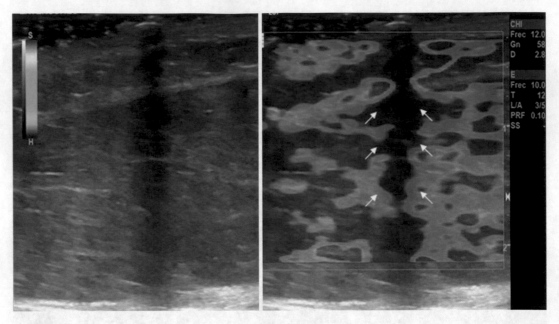

Fig. 5.12 Artifact produced by a gas bubble between the transducer and the skin. Note the shadow on the B mode imaging and the band of increased stiffness in the elastogram (arrows)

- Make sure there are no gas bubbles between the patient and the probe, as they could cause an apparent increase in stiffness (Fig. 5.12).

or predict a given prognosis, and according to such knowledge, introduce elastography in clinical guidelines.

5.4 Conclusion and Future Perspectives

As has been exhibited in this chapter, elastography has great potential to enter clinical practice in diverse scenarios, soon it will be more available in diagnostic facilities and, its results have been demonstrated to be reproducible. Nevertheless, there is still a trip to go. A limitation in the current literature is the lack of large series establishing normality thresholds, which limits the usability of this technique in daily routine. Standardization is a must in the process of achieving this goal, and it will necessarily need to take into account the sonographer's preparation and experience, patient positioning, US probe positioning, previous physical activity in the evaluated patient, muscles to be evaluated, and the unit of measurement. The next step will be to put elastography into the context of diseases and see how such findings can influence the treatment

References

1. Sconfienza LM, Albano D, Allen G, et al. Clinical indications for musculoskeletal ultrasound updated in 2017 by European Society of Musculoskeletal Radiology (ESSR) consensus. Eur Radiol. 2018;28:5338–51.
2. Pillen S, van Alfen N. Skeletal muscle ultrasound. Neurol Res. 2011;33:1016–24.
3. Ryan M, Bisset L, Newsham-West R. Should we care about tendon structure? The disconnect between structure and symptoms in tendinopathy. J Orthop Sports Phys Ther. 2015;45:823–5.
4. Docking SI, Ooi CC, Connell D. Tendinopathy: Is imaging telling us the entire story? J Orthop Sports Phys Ther. 2015;45:842–52.
5. Cosgrove D, Piscaglia F, Bamber J, et al. EFSUMB guidelines and recommendations on the clinical use of ultrasound elastography. Part 2: Clinical applications. Ultraschall Med. 2013;34: 238–53.
6. Harmon B, Wells M, Park D, Gao J. Ultrasound elastography in neuromuscular and movement disorders. Clin Imaging. 2019;53:35–42.
7. Creze M, Nordez A, Soubeyrand M, Rocher L, Maître X, Bellin M-F. Shear wave sonoelastography of skel-

etal muscle: basic principles, biomechanical concepts, clinical applications, and future perspectives. Skelet Radiol. 2018;47:457–71.

8. Cortez CD, Hermitte L, Ramain A, Mesmann C, Lefort T, Pialat JB. Ultrasound shear wave velocity in skeletal muscle: a reproducibility study. Diagn Interv Imaging. 2016;97:71–9.

9. Chapter 5: Muscle: anatomy, physiology, and biochemistry. Firestein & Kelley's textbook of rheumatology. Elsevier; 2021. p. 67–79.

10. Eby SF, Song P, Chen S, Chen Q, Greenleaf JF, An K-N. Validation of shear wave elastography in skeletal muscle. J Biomech. 2013;46:2381–7.

11. Shinohara M, Sabra K, Gennisson J-L, Fink M, Tanter M. Real-time visualization of muscle stiffness distribution with ultrasound shear wave imaging during muscle contraction. Muscle Nerve. 2010;42:438–41.

12. Yoshitake Y, Takai Y, Kanehisa H, Shinohara M. Muscle shear modulus measured with ultrasound shear-wave elastography across a wide range of contraction intensity. Muscle Nerve. 2014;50:103–13.

13. Wang C-Z, Li T-J, Zheng Y-P. Shear modulus estimation on vastus intermedius of elderly and young females over the entire range of isometric contraction. PLoS One. 2014;9:e101769.

14. Eby SF, Cloud BA, Brandenburg JE, Giambini H, Song P, Chen S, LeBrasseur NK, An K-N. Shear wave elastography of passive skeletal muscle stiffness: influences of sex and age throughout adulthood. Clin Biomech (Bristol Avon). 2015;30:22–7.

15. Miyamoto N, Hirata K, Kanehisa H, Yoshitake Y. Validity of measurement of shear modulus by ultrasound shear wave elastography in human pennate muscle. PLoS One. 2015;10:e0124311.

16. Alfuraih AM, O'Connor P, Hensor E, Tan AL, Emery P, Wakefield RJ. The effect of unit, depth, and probe load on the reliability of muscle shear wave elastography: variables affecting reliability of SWE. J Clin Ultrasound. 2018;46:108–15.

17. Botar Jid C, Vasilescu D, Damian L, Dumitriu D, Ciurea A, Dudea SM. Musculoskeletal sonoelastography. Pictorial essay. Med Ultrason. 2012;14:239–45.

18. Winn N, Lalam R, Cassar-Pullicino V. Sonoelastography in the musculoskeletal system: current role and future directions. World J Radiol. 2016;8:868–79.

19. Schleip R, Jäger H, Klingler W. What is "fascia"? A review of different nomenclatures. J Bodyw Mov Ther. 2012;16:496–502.

20. Fascia glossary of terms - Fascia Research Society. https://www.fasciaresearchsociety.org/fascia_glossary_of_terms.php. Accessed 6 Oct 2022.

21. Akagi R, Takahashi H. Acute effect of static stretching on hardness of the gastrocnemius muscle. Med Sci Sports Exerc. 2013;45:1348–54.

22. Akagi R, Yamashita Y, Ueyasu Y. Age-related differences in muscle shear moduli in the lower extremity. Ultrasound Med Biol. 2015;41:2906–12.

23. Bouillard K, Jubeau M, Nordez A, Hug F. Effect of vastus lateralis fatigue on load sharing between quad-riceps femoris muscles during isometric knee extensions. J Neurophysiol. 2014;111:768–76.

24. Alfuraih AM, O'Connor P, Tan AL, Hensor E, Emery P, Wakefield RJ. An investigation into the variability between different shear wave elastography systems in muscle. Med Ultrason. 2017;19:392–400.

25. Paramalingam S, Needham M, Raymond W, Mastaglia F, Lightowler D, Morin N, Counsel P, Keen HI. Muscle shear wave elastography, conventional B mode and power Doppler ultrasonography in healthy adults and patients with autoimmune inflammatory myopathies: a pilot cross-sectional study. BMC Musculoskelet Disord. 2021;22:537.

26. Rosskopf AB, Ehrmann C, Buck FM, Gerber C, Flück M, Pfirrmann CWA. Quantitative shear-wave US elastography of the supraspinatus muscle: reliability of the method and relation to tendon integrity and muscle quality. Radiology. 2016;278:465–74.

27. Amato AA, Barohn RJ. Evaluation and treatment of inflammatory myopathies. J Neurol Neurosurg Psychiatry. 2009;80:1060–8.

28. Mariampillai K, Granger B, Amelin D, et al. Development of a new classification system for idiopathic inflammatory myopathies based on clinical manifestations and myositis-specific autoantibodies. JAMA Neurol. 2018;75:1528–37.

29. Botar-Jid C, Damian L, Dudea SM, Vasilescu D, Rednic S, Badea R. The contribution of ultrasonography and sonoelastography in assessment of myositis. Med Ultrason. 2010;12:120–6.

30. Song Y, Lee S, Yoo DH, Jang K-S, Bae J. Strain sonoelastography of inflammatory myopathies: comparison with clinical examination, magnetic resonance imaging and pathologic findings. Br J Radiol. 2016;89:20160283.

31. Cardamone M, Darras BT, Ryan MM. Inherited myopathies and muscular dystrophies. Semin Neurol. 2008;28:250–9.

32. Cornelson SM, Ruff AN, Perillat M, Kettner NW. Sonoelastography of the trunk and lower extremity muscles in a case of Duchenne muscular dystrophy. J Ultrasound. 2021;24:343–7.

33. Lacourpaille L, Gross R, Hug F, Guével A, Péréon Y, Magot A, Hogrel J-Y, Nordez A. Effects of Duchenne muscular dystrophy on muscle stiffness and response to electrically-induced muscle contraction: a 12-month follow-up. Neuromuscul Disord NMD. 2017;27:214–20.

34. Bromham N, Dworzynski K, Eunson P, Fairhurst C. Cerebral palsy in adults: summary of NICE guidance. BMJ. 2019;364:l806.

35. Graham HK, Rosenbaum P, Paneth N, et al. Cerebral palsy. Nat Rev Dis Primer. 2016;2:1–25.

36. Brandenburg JE, Eby SF, Song P, Kingsley-Berg S, Bamlet W, Sieck GC, An K-N. Quantifying passive muscle stiffness in children with and without cerebral palsy using ultrasound shear wave elastography. Dev Med Child Neurol. 2016;58:1288–94.

37. Lee SSM, Gaebler-Spira D, Zhang L-Q, Rymer WZ, Steele KM. Use of shear wave ultrasound elastogra-

phy to quantify muscle properties in cerebral palsy. Clin Biomech (Bristol Avon). 2016;31:20–8.

38. Vola EA, Albano M, Di Luise C, Servodidio V, Sansone M, Russo S, Corrado B, Servodio Iammarrone C, Caprio MG, Vallone G. Use of ultrasound shear wave to measure muscle stiffness in children with cerebral palsy. J Ultrasound. 2018;21:241–7.

39. Dağ N, Cerit MN, Şendur HN, Zinnuroğlu M, Muşmal BN, Cindil E, Oktar SÖ. The utility of shear wave elastography in the evaluation of muscle stiffness in patients with cerebral palsy after botulinum toxin A injection. J Med Ultrason. 2020;47:609–15.

40. Brandenburg JE, Eby SF, Song P, Bamlet WR, Sieck GC, An K-N. Quantifying effect of onabotulinum toxin A on passive muscle stiffness in children with cerebral palsy using ultrasound shear wave elastography. Am J Phys Med Rehabil. 2018;97:500–6.

41. Paoletta M, Moretti A, Liguori S, Snichelotto F, Menditto I, Toro G, Gimigliano F, Iolascon G. Ultrasound imaging in sport-related muscle injuries: pitfalls and opportunities. Medicina (Mex). 2021;57:1040.

42. Drakonaki EE, Sudoł-Szopińska I, Sinopidis C, Givissis P. High resolution ultrasound for imaging complications of muscle injury: is there an additional role for elastography? J Ultrason. 2019;19:137–44.

43. Martínez-Rodríguez R, Galán-Del-Río F, Cantalapiedra JA, Flórez-García MT, Martínez-Martín J, Álvaro-Meca A, Koppenhaver SL, Fernández-de-Las-Peñas C. Reliability and discriminative validity of real-time ultrasound elastography in the assessment of tissue stiffness after calf muscle injury. J Bodyw Mov Ther. 2021;28:463–9.

44. Zhou J, Lin Y, Zhang J, Si'tu X, Wang J, Pan W, Wang Y. Reliability of shear wave elastography for the assessment of gastrocnemius fascia elasticity in healthy individual. Sci Rep. 2022;12:8698.

45. Kawai T. Shear wave elastography for chronic musculoskeletal problem. London: IntechOpen; 2022. https://doi.org/10.5772/intechopen.102024.

46. Hallén A, Ekstrand J. Return to play following muscle injuries in professional footballers. J Sports Sci. 2014;32:1229–36.

47. Waterworth G, Wein S, Gorelik A, Rotstein AH. MRI assessment of calf injuries in Australian Football League players: findings that influence return to play. Skelet Radiol. 2017;46:343–50.

48. Comin J, Malliaras P, Baquie P, Barbour T, Connell D. Return to competitive play after hamstring injuries involving disruption of the central tendon. Am J Sports Med. 2013;41:111–5.

49. Yoshida K, Itoigawa Y, Maruyama Y, Kaneko K. Healing process of gastrocnemius muscle injury on ultrasonography using B-mode imaging, power Doppler imaging, and shear wave elastography. J Ultrasound Med. 2019;38:3239–46.

50. Zhou X, Wang C, Qiu S, Mao L, Chen F, Chen S. Noninvasive assessment of changes in muscle injury by ultrasound shear wave elastography: an experimental study in contusion model. Ultrasound Med Biol. 2018;44:2759–67.

51. Niitsu M, Michizaki A, Endo A, Takei H, Yanagisawa O. Muscle hardness measurement by using ultrasound elastography: a feasibility study. Acta Radiol. 2011;52:99–105.

52. Akagi R, Tanaka J, Shikiba T, Takahashi H. Muscle hardness of the triceps brachii before and after a resistance exercise session: a shear wave ultrasound elastography study. Acta Radiol. 2015;56:1487–93.

53. Agten CA, Buck FM, Dyer L, Flück M, Pfirrmann CWA, Rosskopf AB. Delayed-onset muscle soreness: temporal assessment with quantitative MRI and shear-wave ultrasound elastography. Am J Roentgenol. 2017;208:402–12.

54. Cummings M, Baldry P. Regional myofascial pain: diagnosis and management. Best Pract Res Clin Rheumatol. 2007;21:367–87.

55. Sikdar S, Shah JP, Gebreab T, Yen R-H, Gilliams E, Danoff J, Gerber LH. Novel applications of ultrasound technology to visualize and characterize myofascial trigger points and surrounding soft tissue. Arch Phys Med Rehabil. 2009;90:1829–38.

56. Ertekin E, Kasar ZS, Turkdogan FT. Is early diagnosis of myofascial pain syndrome possible with the detection of latent trigger points by shear wave elastography? Pol J Radiol. 2021;86:e425–31.

57. Celik D, Mutlu EK. Clinical implication of latent myofascial trigger point. Curr Pain Headache Rep. 2013;17:353.

58. Valera-Calero JA, Sánchez-Jorge S, Buffet-García J, Varol U, Gallego-Sendarrubias GM, Álvarez-González J. Is shear-wave elastography a clinical severity indicator of myofascial pain syndrome? An observational study. J Clin Med. 2021;10:2895.

59. Dieterich AV, Haueise A, Gizzi L. Feeling stiff…but what does it mean objectively?: can you measure muscle tension? Schmerz Berl Ger. 2022;36:242–7.

60. Via AG, Oliva F, Spoliti M, Maffulli N. Acute compartment syndrome. Muscles Ligaments Tendons J. 2015;5:18–22.

61. Hammerberg EM, Whitesides TE, Seiler JG. The reliability of measurement of tissue pressure in compartment syndrome. J Orthop Trauma. 2012;26:24–31; discussion 32.

62. Zhang J, Zhang W, Zhou H, Sang L, Liu L, Sun Y, Gong X, Guan H, Yu M. An exploratory study of two-dimensional shear-wave elastography in the diagnosis of acute compartment syndrome. BMC Surg. 2021;21:418.

63. Irving DB, Cook JL, Young MA, Menz HB. Impact of chronic plantar heel pain on health-related quality of life. J Am Podiatr Med Assoc. 2008;98:283–9.

64. Rompe JD. Plantar fasciopathy. Sports Med Arthrosc Rev. 2009;17:100–4.

65. Wearing SC, Smeathers JE, Urry SR, Hennig EM, Hills AP. The pathomechanics of plantar fasciitis. Sports Med Auckl NZ. 2006;36:585–611.

66. Wu C-H, Chiu Y-H, Chang K-V, Wu W-T, Özçakar L. Ultrasound elastography for the evaluation of plan-

tar fasciitis: a systematic review and meta-analysis. Eur J Radiol. 2022;155:110495.

67. Cruz-Jentoft AJ, Baeyens JP, Bauer JM, et al. Sarcopenia: European consensus on definition and diagnosis. Age Ageing. 2010;39:412–23.

68. Cruz-Jentoft AJ, Bahat G, Bauer J, et al. Sarcopenia: revised European consensus on definition and diagnosis. Age Ageing. 2019;48:16–31.

69. Morley JE. Sarcopenia: diagnosis and treatment. J Nutr Health Aging. 2008;12:452.

70. Chianca V, Albano D, Messina C, Gitto S, Ruffo G, Guarino S, Del Grande F, Sconfienza LM. Sarcopenia: imaging assessment and clinical application. Abdom Radiol N Y. 2022;47:3205–16.

71. Dn P, Pc O, Ej A, Ks N. Comparison of techniques to estimate total body skeletal muscle mass in people of different age groups. Am J Phys. 1999;277:E489. https://doi.org/10.1152/ajpendo.1999.277.3.E489.

72. Prado CMM, Heymsfield SB. Lean tissue imaging: a new era for nutritional assessment and intervention. JPEN J Parenter Enteral Nutr. 2014;38:940–53.

73. Wang J-C, Wu W-T, Chang K-V, Chen L-R, Chi S-Y, Kara M, Özçakar L. Ultrasound imaging for the diagnosis and evaluation of sarcopenia: an umbrella review. Life. 2021;12:9.

74. Bastijns S, De Cock A-M, Vandewoude M, Perkisas S. Usability and pitfalls of shear-wave elastography for evaluation of muscle quality and its potential in assessing sarcopenia: a review. Ultrasound Med Biol. 2020;46:2891–907.

75. Dillman JR, Chen S, Davenport MS, Zhao H, Urban MW, Song P, Watcharotone K, Carson PL. Superficial ultrasound shear wave speed measurements in soft and hard elasticity phantoms: repeatability and reproducibility using two ultrasound systems. Pediatr Radiol. 2015;45:376–85.

76. Kot BCW, Zhang ZJ, Lee AWC, Leung VYF, Fu SN. Elastic modulus of muscle and tendon with shear wave ultrasound elastography: variations with different technical settings. PLoS One. 2012;7:e44348.

77. Liu J, Qian Z, Wang K, Wu J, Jabran A, Ren L, Ren L. Non-invasive quantitative assessment of muscle force based on ultrasonic shear wave elastography. Ultrasound Med Biol. 2019;45:440–51.

78. Andonian P, Viallon M, Goff CL, de Bourguignon C, Tourel C, Morel J, Giardini G, Gergelé L, Millet GP, Croisille P. Shear-wave elastography assessments of quadriceps stiffness changes prior to, during and after prolonged exercise: a longitudinal study during an extreme mountain ultra-marathon. PLoS One. 2016;11:e0161855.

79. Davis LC, Baumer TG, Bey MJ, van Holsbeeck M. Clinical utilization of shear wave elastography in the musculoskeletal system. Ultrasonography. 2019;38:2–12.

Peripheral Nerves

6

Mohamed Abdelmohsen Bedewi

6.1 Introduction

Shear wave elastography (SWE) has been used for the musculoskeletal system. Most studies are focusing on tendons and muscles, however, fewer of them were implemented on peripheral nerves [1]. The basic component of a peripheral nerve is the axon. It is surrounded by the endoneurium which is a connective tissue layer. The perineurium, surrounds multiple axons to form what is called fascicle. Fascicles are surrounded by epineurium which contains blood vessels, fibroblasts and collagen fibers. This anatomic complexity reinforces peripheral nerves with viscoelastic and resistive nature protecting them from mechanical trauma [2]. Studying the mechanical properties of nerves is meant to improve assessment of nerve impairment [3]. Electrodiagnostic tests are considered a reliable method for the diagnosis of peripheral nerve disorders as they provide information about the functional status of neurons. In addition to poor localization, this technique is painful due to needle insertion, takes a long time, and is associated with high incidence of false-negative results [4]. Electrodiagnostic tests are efficient in the assessment of large nerve fibers only, small nerve fibers attain reduced myelin content resulting in slow conduction velocities [5]. Magnetic resonance imaging (MRI) is a useful imaging diagnostic tool with ability to demonstrate excellent topographic anatomy of the peripheral nerves, and to differentiate healthy nerves from pathological ones. Fat-suppressed T2-weighted images could detect the injury site of peripheral nerve as hyperintense. As regeneration occurs the nerve will regain its "iso-intensity." Diffuse tensor imaging is a technique that tracks diffusion of water molecules for better differentiation between healthy and injured nerves. In cases of nerve damage, water molecules demonstrate orthogonal diffusion, while healthy nerves appear as linear structures and water molecules diffuse in an anisotropic pattern. Although MRI is a noninvasive technique, it is time consuming and expensive. Claustrophobic patients are also intolerant to MRI [6–8]. The introduction of modern high-resolution ultrasound provided detailed anatomical information to identify structural pathology of the peripheral nerves especially those with superficial location. Doppler and conventional ultrasound were used for long time as an initial approach for evaluation of some peripheral nerve disorders complementing electrodiagnostic testing and clinical phenotyping [9, 10]. One drawback of conventional ultrasound is the inability to accurately depict changes in the architecture and echogenicity of nerve fascicles during the course of acute/chronic diseases limiting its role in the initial diagnosis and follow-up [11]. Disease of

M. A. Bedewi (✉)
College of Medicine Prince Sattam Bin Abdulaziz University, Al-Kharj, Kingdom of Saudi Arabia
e-mail: m.bedewi@psau.edu.sa

© The Author(s), under exclusive license to Springer Nature Switzerland AG 2023
S. Marsico, A. Solano (eds.), *Elastography of the Musculoskeletal System*,
https://doi.org/10.1007/978-3-031-31054-6_6

the peripheral nerves can lead to changes in their biomechanical features [12]. Any change in the elasticity (softness) of a peripheral nerve could reflect underlying pathophysiology [13]. The introduction of ultrasound elastography allowed better evaluation and identification of tissue abnormalities through the evaluation of nerve elasticity/stiffness.

Currently, there are two main sonographic methods for measuring tissue elasticity: strain elastography, where mild pressure pushes the force impulse and evaluate the tissue stiffness. Strain elastography gives an idea about semiquantitative and qualitative values of tissue stiffness. One of the major disadvantages of this technique is that it is operator dependent, and the measurements taken are not standardized. Shear wave elastography is a less operator-dependent method and can allow visualization and documentation of absolute stiffness in kilopascals or meters per second objectively without maneuvering. SWE gives quantitative and reproducible results [14–16]. Despite the relatively strong nature of the perineurium, it attains limited flexibility and under normal conditions it remains stable by maintaining intraneural pressure. In case of swelling, edema increases the pressure inside neurons making nerves more stiff with an impedance of vascularity [17]. In this chapter, we will consider shear wave elastography (SWE) of the peripheral nerves which we consider more superior to strain elastography since the impulse of excitation from the probe is standardized and uniform.

6.2 Factors Influencing Accurate SWE Measurement of the Peripheral Nerves

To obtain accurate elastographic measurement of a peripheral nerve, confounding factors, and technical limitations should be first considered.

6.2.1 Depth of Acquisition and Probe Orientation

The use of ultrasound systems with a different type of probes could yield different elastographic measurements [18, 19]. The orientation of the probe at the time of measurement is thought to influence SWE measurements, higher values are obtained on long axis compared to short axis [20]. The anisotropic nature, heterogeneity, and distinct borders of the peripheral nerves reflect a challenge in the measurement of tissue elasticity, since Young modulus measurements are based on isotropic homogenous nature of tissues. This makes stiffness calculation sensitive to probe orientation [18, 21–24].

6.2.2 Surrounding Anatomy and Relation to Bone

Proximity to hard structures like bone could lead to stiffness changes due to non-homogenous shear wave propagation [25, 26]. Although it is not possible to change this relation to bone, modifying both the position of the patient and transducer could help to decrease its effect [21]. The presence of adjacent structures with fluid content like cysts, arteries, and veins could also influence SWE values [18]. Tendo-ligamentous structures may also falsely change elasticity. For this reason, we recommend to confine the region of interest (ROI) to be not more than 2 mm in diameter, and this would suit most peripheral nerves. ROIs larger than 2 mm diamater will decrease the accuracy of measurements.

6.2.3 Limb Position

Nerve fascicles are less straight in the relaxed position. Increased tension cause nerve straightening with a change in nerve architecture and concomitant alteration in shear wave velocity. Nerves are known to adapt by stretching with different limb positions and as the stretch increases stiffness and shear wave velocity increase [1]. A chronically flexed joint due to spasticity is known to decrease the CSA but would also increase nerve stiffness [27].

6.2.4 Meters/Second or Kilopascal

Peripheral nerves are complex structures with multiple layers and are considered anisotropic. As a result, the calculated shear wave values related to the Young modulus reflect the same heterogeneity with lesser accuracy [14]. The available ultrasound systems measure SWE via either Young's modulus (kPa) or shear wave velocity (SWV) in meters/second (m/s). Although most studies use kPa, the use of SWV in m/s is considered more accurate since kPa measurement is less reliable on heterogeneous tissues like peripheral nerves [22, 28].

6.3   Upper Limb Nerves

6.3.1   Median Nerve

Entrapment of the median in the carpal tunnel of the wrist joint is considered the most common compressive neuropathy of the upper limb. In neuropathy, there is increased pressure inside the neurons with edema and compression of the blood supply. This will lead to decreased compliance or even demyelination. The end result is will be replacement of the connective tissue, fibrosis, and atrophy of the axons. In carpal tunnel syn-

drome (CTS), there is an alteration of nerve perfusion associated with increased pressure in the carpal tunnel. The etiology could be multifactorial, some of them are due to trauma, and others due to chronic diseases [29]. Using SWE the median nerve stiffness is higher in CTS compared to normal individuals. A cut-off value for the normal elasticity of the median nerve at the wrist was suggested by Kantraci et al. to be 40 kPa [30]. A range of (32–42 kPa) is reasonable for the normal range of elasticity in healthy controls. A range between 66.7 kPa and 100 kPa was recorded for the diagnosis of CTS. Because of the variability in estimating the cut-off value, the wrist-to-forearm ratio was suggested as more accurate for the diagnosis of CTS, where the ratio between patients and controls was 2.1–1 [31]. It is of note that the stiffness of the median nerve decreases after treatment of CTS [32]. This improvement in stiffness was shown to precede nerve morphological changes indicating that SWE could be considered a more sensitive measure of recovery than measuring the nerve caliber in cross-sectional area [33] (Fig. 6.1).

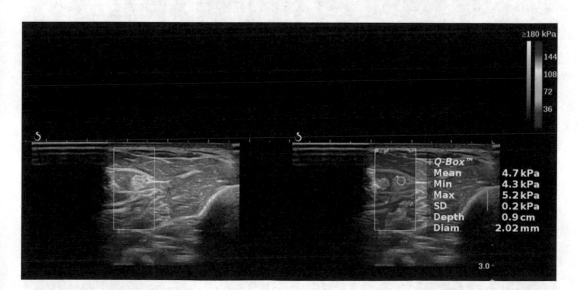

Fig. 6.1 Short-axis view shear wave elastography of the median nerve at the mid-forearm, with minimum, maximum, and mean stiffness in kPa

6.3.2 Ulnar Nerve

Entrapment of the ulnar nerve at the elbow is the second most common neuropathy of the upper limb. The ease of development of neuropathy at this site is attributed to its superficial location making it prone to repetitive irritation, especially in athletes [34]. Compression of the ulnar nerve could lead to high pressure inside the canal with swelling, vascular compromise, and inflammatory changes leading to fibrosis [35]. Some variability is noted between authors regarding the mean stiffness of the ulnar nerve at the cubital tunnel. Paluch et al. reported a mean stiffness of the ulnar nerve at the cubital tunnel to be 33.1 kPa. Interestingly the same group reported a mean stiffness at the forearm to be 49 kPa [36, 37]. Cornelson et al. reported clearly lower stiffness values at the cubital tunnel (11.2 kPa) [38]. The mean SWE stiffness in patients with ulnar neuropathy was 96.38 kPa. Higher stiffness values were reported in the cubital tunnel in patients with ulnar neuropathy compared to the mid-forearm (2.7 versus 1) and distal forearm (2.8 versus 1) [36]. Entrapment of the ulnar nerve at the Guyon's canal also revealed higher stiffness compared to controls (99.41 versus 49 kPa) [37] (Figs. 6.2 and 6.3).

6.3.3 Radial Nerve

One study was found reporting stiffness of the radial nerve in healthy individuals reporting a mean stiffness of 30.3 kPa in the short axis, and 34.9 kPa in the long axis [20]. The difference in elasticity is likely attributed to proximity of the nerve to the humerus in the long axis. One case of a radial nerve schwannoma was studied by Bhatalgia et al. and revealed an elasticity ranging between 24 and 30 kPa which indicates benign nature [39] (Figs. 6.4 and 6.5).

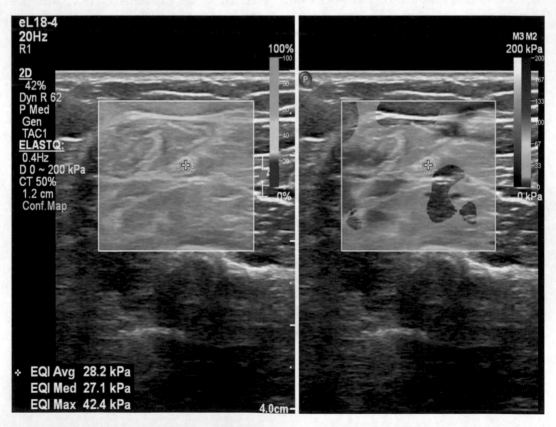

Fig. 6.2 Short-axis view of the ulnar nerve shear wave elastography, with confidence map on the left, color map scale on the right, for measurement of stiffness in kPa

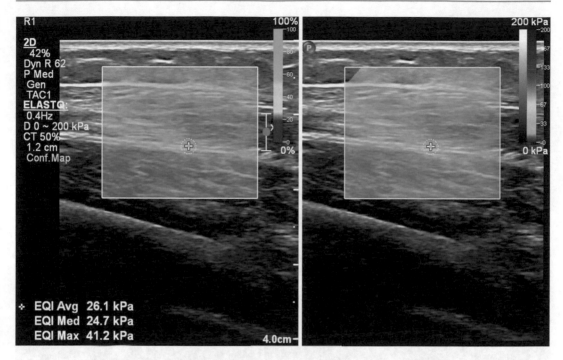

Fig. 6.3 Long-axis view of the ulnar nerve shear wave elastography, with confidence map on the left, color map scale on the right, for measurement of stiffness in kPa

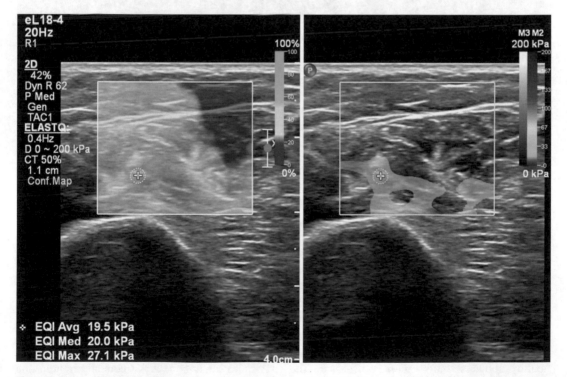

Fig. 6.4 Short-axis view of the radial nerve shear wave elastography (confidence map on left, color map scale on right) for measurement of stiffness in kPa

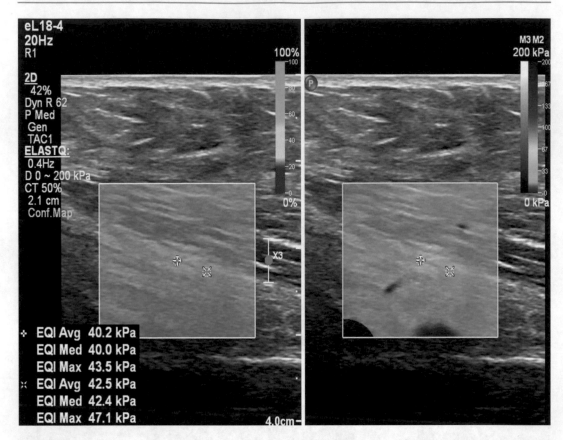

Fig. 6.5 Long-axis view of radial nerve shear wave elastography (confidence map on left, color map scale on right) for measurement of stiffness in kPa

6.4 Lower Limb Nerves

6.4.1 Tibial Nerve

The tibial nerve is the distal and larger extensions of the sciatic nerve which is the largest nerve of the body. Evaluation of the tibial by nerve conduction study (NCS) is considered the main method for the diagnosis of diabetic polyneuropathy (DPN). The mean stiffness of the normal tibial nerve was reported by many authors to range between 26 and 32 kPa [17, 40, 41]. Using SWE, stiffness of the tibial was higher in diabetic patients with DPN compared to healthy subjects. Even diabetic patients without DPN recorded higher stiffness of the tibial nerve compared to healthy subjects. Furthermore, stiffness of the tibial nerve was higher in a category of patients showing clinical features of DPN with negative

results on NCS. The increase in stiffness was proportional to the degree of neuropathy [18, 41]. According to Dikici et al., the tibial nerve stiffness in diabetic neuropathy patients ranges between 59 kPa in the mild form and 81 kPa in the severe form [17]. The aforementioned information suggests the potential ability of SWE to detect DPN on a subclinical basis. The role of SWE in evaluation of neuropathy is enhanced by performing serial follow-up to assess disease progression (Figs. 6.6, 6.7, and 6.8).

6.4.2 Common Fibular Nerve

The common fibular nerve is one of the important lower limb nerves that is frequently injured due to its superficial location. The common fibular nerve is prone to chronic irritation and compres-

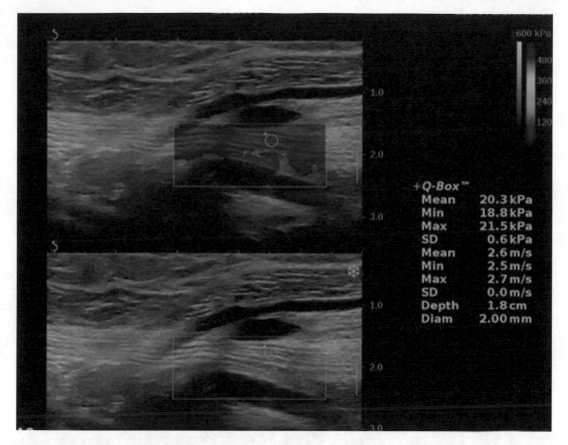

Fig. 6.6 Short-axis view shear wave elastography of the tibial nerve, with color map, minimum, maximum, and mean stiffness in kPa

sion by cast or space-occupying lesions like ganglion cysts. Chen et al. reported a mean stiffness of the common fibular nerve to be 17.2 kPa. Another study group reported a mean stiffness for this nerve in the long axis to be 35 kPa, and in the short axis to be 22.5 kPa [42, 43]. The stiffness of a schwannoma of the common fibular nerve was studied by Cantisani et al. and revealed higher stiffness than the surroundings [44] (Figs. 6.9 and 6.10).

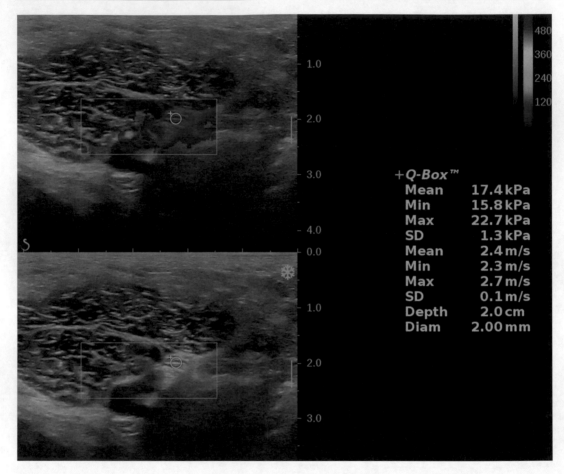

Fig. 6.7 Long-axis view shear wave elastography of the tibial nerve, with color map, minimum, maximum, and mean stiffness in kPa

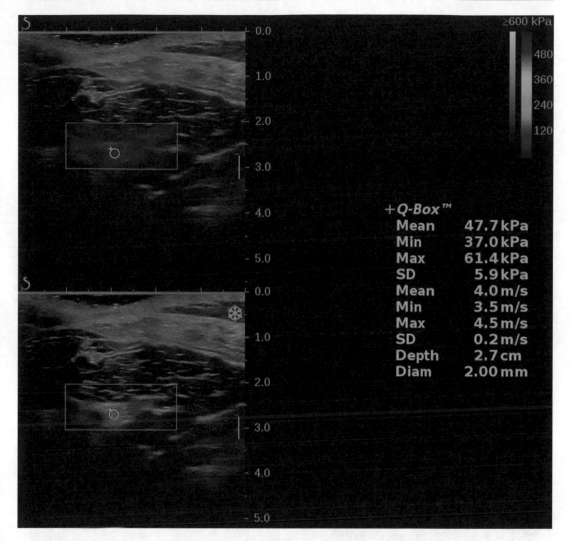

Fig. 6.8 Short-axis view shear wave elastography of the tibial nerve in a Type II diabetic patient with increased stiffness (47.7 kPa)

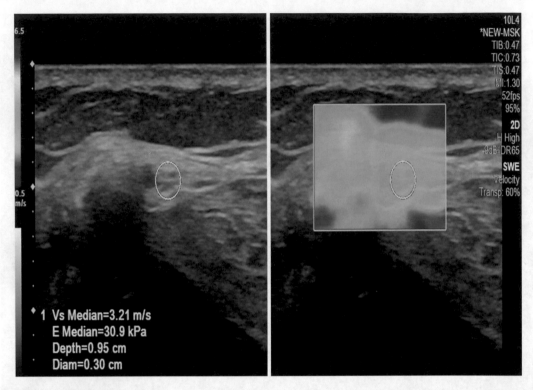

Fig. 6.9 Short-axis view of the common fibular nerve shear wave elastography, with color map scale on the right, and stiffness measurements on the left in both kPa (kilopascals) and meters per second (m/s)

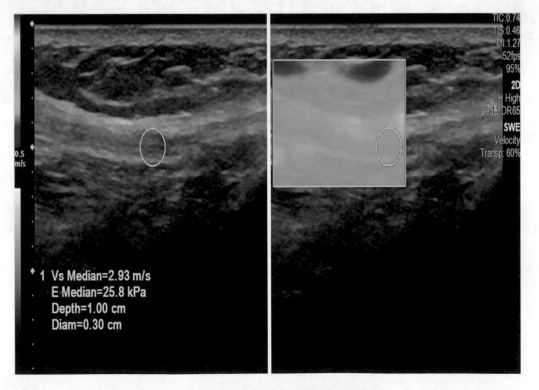

Fig. 6.10 Long-axis view of the common fibular nerve shear wave elastography, with color map scale on the right, and stiffness measurements on the left in both kPa (kilopascals) and meters per second (m/s)

6.5 The Brachial Plexus

SWE of the brachial plexus is challenging due to the complexity of the surrounding anatomy, especially vascular structures, and occasional presence of anatomical variation of the scalene muscles. Another important factor is the lack of typical fascicular pattern of the nerve roots in this area, which makes their identification a difficult task in unexperienced hands. The available studies of the C5–C7 brachial plexus roots reported stiffness values ranging between 13 and 16 kPa [45, 46]. Gurun et al. demonstrated an increase in the stiffness of C5 and C6 roots in patients with multiple sclerosis compared to the control group [47]. Kultur et al. demonstrated increased stiffness of the brachial plexus after radiation therapy for breast malignancy [48] (Fig. 6.11).

A summary of the findings in different clinical conditions can be found in Table 6.1.

Table 6.1 Summary of SWE stiffness findings in some pathologies of peripheral nerves

Disease	Stiffness
Diabetic neuropathy	Increased
Diabetic patient without neuropathy	Increased
Carpal tunnel syndrome	Increased
Ulnar neuropathy	Increased
Neurofibromatosis	Decreased
Leprosy	Increased
Acromegaly	Increased
Systemic sclerosis	Increased
Schwannoma	Equivocal

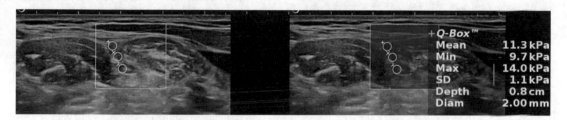

Fig. 6.11 Short-axis view shear wave elastography of the brachial plexus roots at the interscalene groove, with color map, minimum, maximum, and mean stiffness in kPa

6.6   New Horizons in Peripheral Nerve SWE

Recent research revealed increased stiffness of the median nerve in acromegaly, systemic sclerosis, and leprosy [49–51]. Staber et al. suggested a role for SWE in neurofibromatosis. Interestingly, these patients showed lower stiffness than healthy controls [52]. In addition to a role in nerve recovery, a future role of SWE is to guide perineural hydrodissection. This is achieved by identifying areas of nerve entrapment related to scar tissue. In these cases, the fibrous scar tissue causes distortion and adhesions around nerves which are difficult to be identified by conventional ultrasound. SWE will recognize the hard areas related to scars causing neural compression in complicated postoperative cases [53, 54]. Karakaya et al. assessed the stiffness of the sciatic nerve after nerve block and suggested a role for SWE to help give quantitative information about success of the nerve block by measuring stiffness of the sciatic nerve before and after injection of the local anesthetic [55].

6.7   Conclusion

SWE is a promising diagnostic tool that is gaining more popularity in the assessment of peripheral nerves. We believe that it could complement electrodiagnostic tools and clinical phenotyping. More structured studies are still needed to increase the validity and reliability of measurements.

References

1. Greening J, Dilley A. Posture-induced changes in peripheral nerve stiffness measured by ultrasound shear-wave elastography. Muscle Nerve. 2017;55:213–22.
2. Zhu B, Yan F, He Y, Wang L, Xiang X, Tang Y, Yang Y, Qiu L. Evaluation of the healthy median nerve elasticity: feasibility and reliability of shear wave elastography. Medicine (Baltimore). 2018 Oct;97(43):e12956.
3. Rugel CL, Franz CK, Lee SSM. Influence of limb position on assessment of nerve mechanical properties using shear wave ultrasound elastography. Muscle Nerve. 2020;61:616–22.
4. Tang X, Zhu B, Tian M, Guo R, Huang S, Tang Y, Qiu L. Preliminary study on the influencing factors of shear wave elastography for peripheral nerves in healthy population. Sci Rep. 2021;11(1):5582.
5. Terkelsen AJ, Karlsson P, Lauria G, et al. The diagnostic challenge of small fiber neuropathy: clinical presentations, evaluations, and causes. Lancet Neurol. 2017;16:934–44.
6. Rangavajla G, Mokarram N, Masoodzadehgan N, Pai SB, Bellamkonda RV. Noninvasive imaging of peripheral nerves. Cells Tissues Organs. 2014;200(1):69–77.
7. Tagliafico A, Bignotti B, Tagliafico G, Martinoli C. Peripheral nerve MRI: precision and reproducibility of T2*- derived measurements at 3.0-T: a feasibility study. Skeletal Radiol. 2015;44(5):679–86.
8. Aggarwal A, Jana M, Srivastava DN, Sharma R, Gamanagatti S, Kumar A, et al. Magnetic resonance neurography and ultrasonogram findings in upper limb peripheral neuropathies. Neurol India. 2019;67(Supplement):S125–34.
9. Taljanovic MS, Gimber LH, Becker GW, et al. Shear-wave elastography: basic physics and musculoskeletal applications. Radiographics. 2017;37(3):855–70.
10. Hannaford A, Vucic S, Kiernan MC, Simon NG. Review Article: "Spotlight on ultrasonography in the diagnosis of peripheral nerve disease: the evidence to date". Int J Gen Med. 2021;14:4579–604.
11. Van Hooren B, Teratsias P, Hodson-Tole EF. Ultrasound imaging to assess skeletal muscle architecture during movements: a systematic review of methods, reliability, and challenges. J Appl Physiol. 2020;128(4):978–99.
12. Ryu JA, Jeong WK. Current status of musculoskeletal application of shear wave elastography. Ultrasonography. 2017;36:185–97.
13. Klauser AS, Miyamoto H, Bellmann-Weiler R, Feuchtner GM, Wick MC, Jaschke WR. Sonoelastography: musculoskeletal applications. Radiology. 2014;272(3):622–33.
14. Shiina T, Nightingale KR, Palmeri ML, et al. WFUMB guidelines and recommendations for clinical use of ultrasound elastography. Part 1: basic principles and terminology. Ultrasound Med Biol. 2015;41(5):1126–47.
15. Hobson-Webb LD. Emerging technologies in neuromuscular ultrasound. Muscle Nerve. 2020;61:719–25.
16. Winn N, Lalam R, Cassar-Pullicino V. Sonoelastography in the musculoskeletal system: current role and future directions. World J Radiol. 2016;8:868–79.
17. Dikici AS, Ustabasioglu FE, Delil S, et al. Evaluation of the tibial nerve with shear-wave elastography: a potential sonographic method for the diagnosis of diabetic peripheral neuropathy. Radiology. 2017;282:494–501.
18. Wee TC, Simon NG. Ultrasound elastography for the evaluation of peripheral nerves: a systematic review. Muscle Nerve. 2019;60:501–12.

19. Dillman JR, Chen S, Davenport MS, et al. Superficial ultrasound shear wave speed measurements in soft and hard elasticity phantoms: repeatability and reproducibility using two ultrasound systems. Pediatr Radiol. 2015;45(3):376–85.

20. Bedewi MA, Kotb MA, Aldossary NM, Abodonya AM, Saleh AK. Swify SM Shear wave elastography of the radial nerve in healthy subjects. J Int Med Res. 2021;49(1):300060520987938.

21. Davis LC, Baumer TG, Bey MJ, et al. Clinical utilization of shear wave elastography in the musculoskeletal system. Ultrasonography. 2019;38:2–12.

22. Alfuraih AM, O'Connor P, Hensor E, Tan AL, Emery P, Wakefield RJ. The effect of unit, depth, and probe load on the reliability of muscle shear wave elastography: variables affecting reliability of SWE. J Clin Ultrasound. 2018;46(2):108–15.

23. Shin HJ, Kim MJ, Kim HY, Roh YH, Lee MJ. Comparison of shear wave velocities on ultrasound elastography between different machines, transducers, and acquisition depths: a phantom study. Eur Radiol. 2016;26(10):3361–7.

24. Mulabecirovic A, Vesterhus M, Gilja OH, Havre RF. In vitro comparison of five different elastography systems for clinical applications,using strain and shear wave technology. Ultrasound Med Biol. 2016;42(11):2572–88.

25. Zakrzewski J, Zakrzewska K, Pluta K, et al. Ultrasound elastography in the evaluation of peripheral neuropathies: a systematic review of theliterature. Pol J Radiol. 2019;84:e581–91.

26. Bortolotto C, Turpini E, Felisaz P, et al. Median nerve evaluation by shear wave elastosonography: impact of "bone-proximity" hardening artifacts and inter-observer agreement. J Ultrasound. 2017;20:293–9.

27. Aslan H, Analan PD. Effects of chronic flexed wrist posture on the elasticity and crosssectional area of the median nerve at the carpal tunnel among chronic stroke patients. Med Ultrason. 2018;1(1):71–5.

28. Youk JH, Son EJ, Park AY, Kim JA. Shear-wave elastography for breast masses: local shear wave speed (m/sec) versus Young modulus (kPa). Ultrasonography. 2014;33:34–9.

29. Dąbrowska-Thing A, Zakrzewski J, Nowak O, Nitek Ż. Ultrasound elastography as a potential method to evaluate entrapment neuropathies in elite athletes: a mini-review. Pol J Radiol. 2019;84:e625–9.

30. Kantarci F, Ustabasioglu FE, Delil S, et al. Median nerve stiffness measurement by shear wave elastography: a potential sonographic method in the diagnosis of carpal tunnel syndrome. Eur Radiol. 2014;24:434–40.

31. Paluch Ł, Pietruski P, Walecki J, et al. Wrist to forearm ratio as a median nerve shear wave elastography test in carpal tunnel syndrome diagnosis. J Plast Reconstr Aesthet Surg. 2018;71:1146–52.

32. Asadov R, Erdal A, Bugdaycı O, Gündüz OH, Ekinci G. The effectiveness of ultrasonography and ultrasonographic elastography in the diagnosis of carpal tunnel syndrome and evaluation of treatment response after steroid injection. Eur J Radiol. 2018;108:172–6.

33. Yoshii Y, Tung WL, Ishii T. Strain and morphological changes of median nerve after carpal tunnel release. J Ultrasound Med. 2017;36(6):1153–9.

34. Brubacher JW, Leversedge FJ. Ulnar neuropathy in cyclists. Hand Clin. 2017;33:199–205.

35. Kim S, Lee GY. Evaluation of the ulnar nerve with shear-wave elastography: a potential sonographic method for the diagnosis of ulnar neuropathy. Ultrasonography. 2021;40(3):349–56.

36. Paluch Ł, Noszczyk B, Nitek Ż, et al. Shear-wave elastography: a new potential method to diagnose ulnar neuropathy at the elbow. Eur Radiol. 2018;28:4932–9.

37. Paluch Ł, Noszczyk BH, Walecki J, et al. Shear-wave elastography in the diagnosis of ulnar tunnel syndrome. J Plast Reconstr Aesthet Surg. 2018;71:1593–9.

38. Cornelson SM, Sclocco R, Kettner NW. Ulnar nerve instability in the cubital tunnel of asymptomatic volunteers. J Ultrasound. 2019;22:337–44.

39. Battaglia PJ, Carbone-Hobbs V, Guebert GM, et al. High-resolution ultrasonography and shear-wave sonoelastography of a cystic radial nerve Schwannoma. J Ultrasound. 2017;20:261–6.

40. Bedewi MA, Elsifey AA, Alfaifi T, Kotb MA, Abdelgawad MS, Bediwy AM, Swify SM, Awad EM. Shear wave elastography of the tibial nerve in healthy subjects. Medicine (Baltimore). 2021;100(3):e23999.

41. Jiang W, Huang S, Teng H, et al. Diagnostic performance of two dimensional shear wave elastography for evaluating tibial nerve stiffness in patients with diabetic peripheral neuropathy. Eur Radiol. 2019;29:2167–74.

42. Chen R, Wang XL, Xue WL, et al. Application value of conventional ultrasound and real-time shear wave elastography in patients with type 2 diabetic polyneuropathy. Eur J Radiol. 2020;126:108965.

43. Bedewi MA, Alhariqi BA, Aldossary NM, Gaballah AH, Sandougah KJ, Kotb MA. Shear wave elastography of the common fibular nerve at the fibular head. Medicine (Baltimore). 2022;101(11):e29052.

44. Cantisani V, Orsogna N, Porfiri A, Fioravanti C, D'Ambrosio F. Elastographic and contrast-enhanced ultrasound features of a benign schwannoma of the common fibular nerve. J Ultrasound. 2013;16:135–8.

45. Bedewi MA, Nissman D, Aldossary NM, Maetani TH, ElSharkawy MS, Koura H. Shear wave elastography of the brachial plexus roots at the interscalene groove. Neurol Res. 2018;40(9):805–10.

46. Aslan A, Aktan A, Aslan M, Gulseren Y, Kabaalioglu A. Shear wave and strain elastographic features of the brachial plexus in healthy adults: reliability of the findings-a pilot study. J Ultrasound Med. 2018;35(10):2353–62.

47. Gürün E, Akdulum İ, Akyüz M, Oktar SÖ. Shear wave elastography evaluation of brachial plexus in multiple sclerosis. Acta Radiol. 2022;63(4):520–6.

48. Kültür T, Okumuş M, İnal M, Yalçın S. Evaluation of the brachial plexus with shear wave elastography after

radiotherapy for breast cancer. J Ultrasound Med. 2018;37:2029–35.

49. Burulday V, Dogan A, Sahan MH, Arikan S, Gungunes A. Ultrasound elastography of the median nerve in patients with acromegaly: a case-control study. J Ultrasound Med. 2018;37:2371–7.

50. Yagci I, Kenis-Coskun O, Ozsoy T, Ozen G, Direskeneli H. Increased stiffness of median nerve in systemic sclerosis. BMC Musculoskelet Disord. 2017;18(1):434.

51. Meghashyam K, Prakash M, Narang T, Sinha A, Sandhu MS. Role of shear wave elastography in treatment follow-up of leprosy neuropathy. J Ultrasound. 2022 Jun;25(2):265–72.

52. Staber D, Oppold J, Grimm A, Schuhmann MU, Romano A, Marquetand J, Kleiser B. Shear-wave-elastography in neurofibromatosis type I. Diagnostics (Basel). 2022;12(2):360.

53. Snoj Ž, Wu CH, Taljanovic MS, Dumić-Čule I, Drakonaki EE, Klauser AS. Ultrasound elastography in musculoskeletal radiology: past, present, and future. Semin Musculoskelet Radiol. 2020;24(2):156–66.

54. Su DC, Chang KV, Lam SKH. Shear wave elastography to guide perineural hydrodissection: two case reports. Diagnostics (Basel). 2020;10:348.

55. Karakaya MA, Ince I, Kucukerdem OB, Bas A, Gurkan Y. Assessment of sciatic nerve block success with elastography: new perspective for the nerve blocks. Minerva Anestesiol. 2021;87(12):1380–1381l.

Rheumatological and Joint Pathology

7

Irene Carrión Barberà, Salvatore Marsico,
María Pumar Pérez, Albert Solano,
and Tarek Carlos Salman Monte

7.1   Introduction

Ultrasound (US) is an imaging technique widely used in patients with musculoskeletal diseases to detect signs of inflammation [1]. The diagnostic imaging methods that are currently most used to diagnose synovitis are ultrasound (US), with the use of Power Doppler (PD) [1, 2], and Magnetic Resonance Imaging (MRI), emerging as a potentially useful diagnostic tool in inflammatory pathologies of the musculoskeletal system [3].

In 2017, OMERACT US (Outcome Measures in Rheumatoid Arthritis Clinical Trials Ultrasound) Work Group, published a combined scoring system in rheumatoid arthritis (RA) using both gray scale (GS) and PD ultrasound in RA [4].

In 2021, the European League Against Rheumatism (EULAR) presented recommendations for the reporting of ultrasound studies in musculoskeletal disease. It presents the modalities of ultrasound study and for the first time, elastography is lightly named [5].

In 2020, an article about elastography was published [6] in which the authors stated that it is considered the most important advance in US technology, since Doppler Ultrasound imaging implementation.

In this chapter, we have reviewed the major application of elastosonography in inflammatory and rheumatological pathologies, also evaluating the most interesting perspectives in this field.

I. C. Barberà · T. C. S. Monte
Department of Rheumatology, Hospital del Mar,
Barcelona, Spain

S. Marsico (✉) · M. P. Pérez · A. Solano
Department of Radiology, Hospital del Mar,
Barcelona, Spain
e-mail: 40161@parcdesalutmar.cat

7.2 De Quervain's Tendinopathy

De Quervain's tendinopathy affects the abductor pollicis longus (APL) and extensor pollicis brevis (EPB) tendons in the first extensor compartment at the styloid process of the radius. It is a common cause of wrist pain in adults. It is most common among women aged between 30 and 50 years, including a small subset of women in the postpartum period [7, 8]. Etiopathogenetically it has always been said that it is due to repetitive actions of the first compartment of the finger, but it is not clear, and it may even be that hormonal factors are involved [9]. Diagnosis is made clinically, plain radiography is normal, and ultrasound reveals a thickened extensor retinaculum, hypervascularization on Doppler ultrasound, thickening of the APL and EPB, and partial thinning of the tendon of the EPB due to stenosis by the retinaculum [10]. In relation to treatment, rehabilitation and the use of a hand splint are useful and if there is still no improvement, treatment with steroid anti-inflammatory drugs can be done, followed by infiltration with corticosteroids and if it is very recurrent or there is no improvement, even surgical intervention.

Regarding the SWE findings of De Quervain tenosynovitis, we find in the literature the study of Turkay et al. [11] where 80 patients, 40 healthy controls, and 40 patients with symptomatic De Quervain's tendinitis are included. B-mode ultrasound and SWE to a total number of 80 participants were performed. They found that the median SWE value of the tendon sheath in the healthy group (group 1) was 72 kPa and in the De Quervain patient group (group 2) was 29 kPa. Two groups demonstrated statistically significant differences ($p < 0.001$) so they con-

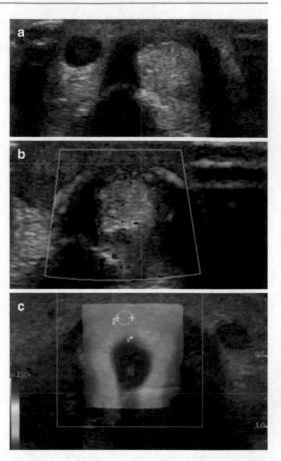

Fig. 7.1 A 51-year-old male patient with persistent pain and swelling localized in the left-hand anatomical snuffbox. Moderate fluid distention of the first extensor tendon compartment sheath was diagnosed with conventional ultrasound (**a**). In the Power Doppler study, the tenosynovial effusion shows a widespread increase in vascularization (**b**). In the SWE study, the tenosynovial effusion does not show high stiffness (**c**). Findings are compatible with De Quervain's tenosynovitis

cluded that SWE modality can provide useful data regarding De Quervain tenosynovitis (Fig. 7.1).

7.3 Systemic Lupus Erythematosus

Systemic lupus erythematosus (SLE) is a systemic autoimmune disease with a wide spectrum of clinical manifestations. It can appear at any age, but most patients begin with symptoms between the ages of 15 and 40 years. The ratio between the female and male genders is 9:1, respectively [12]. SLE is a disease with a universal distribution of 1.8–7.6 cases per 100,000 inhabitants/year in different areas of the USA and from 3.3 to 4.8 cases per 100,000 inhabitants/year in different countries of northern Europe [13–16]. Among the factors mentioned, SLE could be defined as a disease with a predilection for the female sex, especially during the fertile age, and for certain racial groups, such as the black American race or Afro-American and Asian populations. Regarding its etiopathogenic mechanisms, it can be affirmed that SLE is a complex autoimmune disease in which, despite continuous research, there are still many unknowns to be resolved. SLE is characterized by an aberrant autoimmune response, the causes of which have not yet been fully elucidated. Considering a multifactorial cause, traditionally, environmental, and hormonal factors have been postulated that interact with genetic factors that trigger the appearance of an abnormal immune response with an increase in the function of helper T lymphocytes and with the consequent hyperactivity of B lymphocytes and secondary hyperproduction of autoantibodies [17].

As for the clinical manifestations, it is a disease with a multitude of symptoms that affects several organs and systems, the most frequent being the musculoskeletal system, followed by the skin and the kidney [18], but multiple other organs as the heart, lungs, and brain, etc. could be affected and has a wide variety of clinical manifestations and severity, ranging from mild cutaneous involvement or arthralgia to end-stage renal disease, or, for example, central nervous system involvement [19].

As there is no clinical sign or analytical finding or pathognomonic test of SLE, it has been necessary to establish criteria to classify the disease. These criteria are not essential to establish a clinical diagnosis but are used to include patients in different studies and clinical trials. Traditionally, the 1982 ACR classification criteria have been used, and revised, without being validated, in 1997 [20]. Due to the presence of some limitations in these criteria (excessive representation of skin manifestations, impossibility of diagnosing a case of isolated lupus nephropathy confirmed by renal biopsy, without other accompanying symptoms), the SLICC working group has recently proposed new classification criteria in 2012 [21]. Finally, in 2019, ACR and EULAR developed new criteria, which have gained in sensitivity and specificity [22].

Regarding the SWE findings, there is in the literature only a single study evaluating the muscular system in lupus (not the joint). In the study of Di Matteo et al. [23] 30 SLE patients (without previous/current myositis or neuromuscular disorders) and 15 age, sex, and BMI-matched healthy subjects were included. Quadriceps muscle thickness for muscle mass, muscle echogenicity (using a visual semiquantitative scale and gray-scale analysis with histograms) for muscle quality, and SWE for muscle stiffness, were assessed. No difference in the quadriceps muscle thickness was observed between SLE patients and healthy subjects, conversely, muscle echogenicity was significantly increased in SLE patients. Similarly, SWE was significantly lower in SLE patients compared with healthy subjects and muscle echogenicity was inversely correlated with grip strength and SPPB (short physical performance battery) therefore the authors concluded that ultrasound assessment of muscle echogenicity and stiffness is useful for the early detection of muscle involvement in SLE patients.

The literature on the musculoskeletal evaluation of SLE by ultrasound is abundant. However, the heterogeneity of the technique used, the anatomical areas and the patients evaluated is so broad that it is difficult to draw specific conclusions. Thus, a highly variable frequency of synovitis is observed, in 25–94% of patients: wrist 22–94%, MCP 11–84%, proximal IF joint 7–58%, knees 42%, and MTF 50%. The presence of tenosynovitis was reported in 28–65% of patients and as for the erosions, we also found high variability in the different series with a frequency between 2 and 41%. Finally, it is worth noting the high prevalence of subclinical synovitis with frequency variability between 39 and 85% of patients with little or no symptoms in the articular domain [24–26].

7.4 Primary Sjögren's Syndrome

Primary Sjögren's syndrome (pSS) is a systemic autoimmune disease characterized by involvement of the exocrine glands and multisystem involvement, with a prevalence of between 0.1 and 0.6% of the population [27]. It mainly affects women, with a female/male ratio of 9–10:1 [28] and the peak incidence usually appears in the fourth and fifth decades of life, although it can appear at any age. In the Spanish population, the mean age at diagnosis is between 50 and 53 years (range 14–88 years) [29] and only between 9.2 and 15% of patients with SSp are diagnosed at 70 years or older [29, 30]. In other European cohorts, diagnoses of pSS are reported in 6% at the age of 65 years [31].

In addition to glandular involvement, it is also associated with a group of extraglandular manifestations, which are those that will determine the prognosis of the disease (cytopenia, hypergammaglobulinemia or hypocomplementemia, joint, pulmonary, renal, and nervous system involvement, and even lymphoma) [29].

In 2010, EULAR proposed different activity indices: the ESSPRI (EULAR Sjögren's Syndrome Patient Reported Index and the ESSDAI (EULAR Sjögren's syndrome disease activity index scores), which are those used in routine clinical practice [32, 33]. EULAR has recently published EULAR the guidelines for the topical and systemic treatment of pSS [34]. For the classification of the disease, the ACR-EULAR criteria of the year 2017 are followed [35].

There are various studies that have determined different ultrasound classifications in Sjogren's syndrome [36–45] based primarily on glandular size and ultrasound features.

Mainly ecographic scoring systems, from 0 to 3, from 0 to 16, and from 0 to 48, are used, which have different results in terms of diagnostic sensitivity and specificity.

In relation to SWE, there are some advances especially in the diagnosis of glandular involvement [46–48]. In the study by Oruk et al., 49 patients with pSS were studied and compared with 49 healthy controls. The sensitivity, specificity, positive predictive value (PPV), and negative predictive value (NPV) of MSGUS (major salivary gland ultrasonography) and shear wave velocity (SWV) values were investigated. The mean SWV values of the parotid and submandibular glands were significantly higher in pSS patients than in controls ($P < 0.05$). So, the authors concluded that adding SWE to the parotid gland grading system increased the sensitivity and specificity (sensitivity, 82.7%; specificity, 83.7%). They established a cut-off of normal elasticity values in m/s of 2.39 m/s for the parotid gland and 1.95 m/s for the submandibular gland [36]. In the study of Arslan et al. studied 53 patients with pSS and 30 healthy volunteers. The echogenicity of all submandibular and parotid glands was evaluated with B-mode ultrasound, and their elasticity was assessed with 2D SWE (two-dimensional (2D shear wave elastography)). The mean shear wave speed and elasticity mode values for the submandibular and parotid glands were significantly higher in the patients with pSS ($P < 0.05$) therefore their conclusion was that the two-dimensional SWE is an effective technique for assessment of the parenchyma of the salivary glands in patients with pSS and predicts interstitial fibrosis and the severity of histologic damage. They also established a cut-off of normal elasticity values of 2.48 m/s for the parotid gland and 24 kPA for the submandibular gland [37]. Finally, the article by

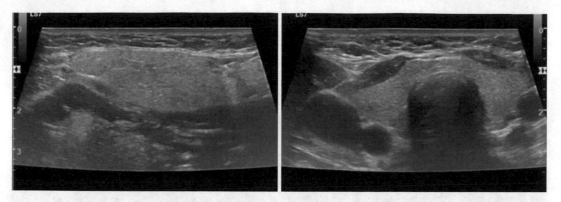

Fig. 7.2 The echogenicity of the submandibular gland (left) should be similar to that of the thyroid gland (right)

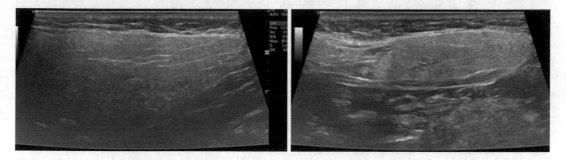

Fig. 7.3 Morphology and normal echogenicity of the parotid (left) and submandibular gland (right) in the sagittal plane

Bădărînză et al. described the usefulness of the shear wave to diagnose cases of lymphoma. The presence of lymphoma within the pSS does not have a specific biomarker and is sometimes difficult to diagnose. The authors concluded that the 2D-SWE had added value for pSS diagnosis in cases where GSUS (GS-US) aspect is normal or nonspecific, the increased stiffness of parotid NHL (non-Hodgkin lymphoma) could be used for early diagnosis, biopsy guidance, and possibly for follow-up and treatment [46] (Figs. 7.2, 7.3, 7.4, 7.5, and 7.6).

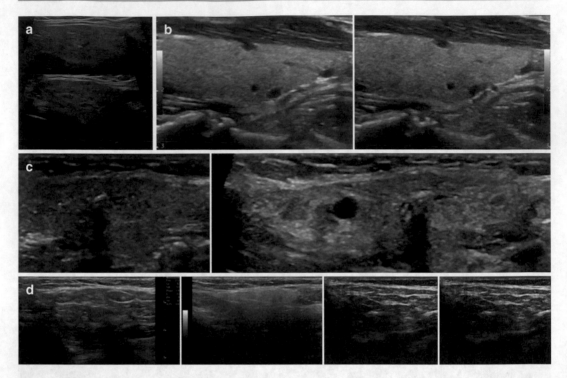

Fig. 7.4 Characteristic ultrasonographic finding in Sjogren's syndrome. (**a, b**) Alteration of the ultrasonographic structure of the submandibular glandS by the presence of small, non-confluent hypoechoic images. (**c**) Alteration of ultrasound structure of the submandibular gland with decreased generalized echogenicity associated with scattered calcifications. (**d**) Alteration of the parotid gland with a generalized decrease in echogenicity and alteration of the echostructure without being able to define in this case the presence of focal hypoechoic intraglandular lesions

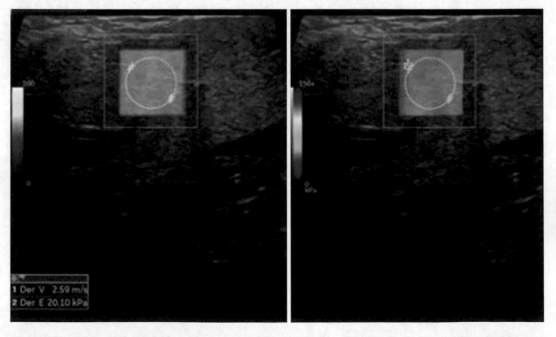

Fig. 7.5 Alteration of echogenicity and SWE values obtained from the submandibular glands in a 56-year-old female patient with Sjogren's syndrome

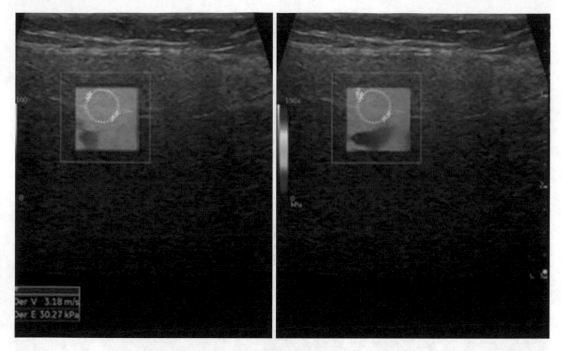

Fig. 7.6 Alteration of echogenicity and SWE values obtained from the study of the parotid glands in a 39-year-old male patient with Sjogren's syndrome

7.5   Gout

Gout is a common condition caused by the deposition of monosodium urate crystals in articular and nonarticular structures. It presents as intermittent episodes of severely painful arthritis (gout flares) caused by the innate immune response to deposited monosodium urate crystals. The typical first presentation of gout is an intensely painful acute inflammatory arthritis affecting a lower limb joint, typically self-limiting over a period of 7–14 days. After resolution, there is a pain-free asymptomatic period (intercritical gout), until another gout flare occurs. Over time, some people with persistent hyperuricemia also develop tophi, chronic gouty arthritis (GA), and structural joint damage.

Gout flares can occur in the joints or periarticular tissues (e.g., bursae, tendons, and entheses). Another well-described feature is its short time from onset to peak intensity (usually less than 12 h) and accompanying features of the flare consisting of swelling, warmth, erythema, and substantial limitation in the ability to use the affected area.

Lower limbs (foot, ankle, and knee) are preferentially involved, while the involvement of the first metatarsophalangeal joint (podagra) is characteristic. Gout flares can also occur in the elbows, wrists, and hand joints, but upper limb involvement usually occurs only in patients with long-standing, poorly controlled disease. Involvement of the axial skeleton occurs occasionally. Gout flares are usually monoarticular, although oligoarticular or polyarticular episodes do occur, typically in patients with a poorly controlled disease or during hospitalization. Polyarticular flares can be associated with pronounced systemic symptoms.

Manifestations of long-standing disease without adequate serum urate control include subcutaneous tophi present as draining or chalk-like subcutaneous nodules under transparent skin, often with overlying vascularity, located in typical locations: joints, ears, olecranon bursae, finger pads, tendons (e.g., Achilles). Joint deformity and associated joint damage are common in patients with tophaceous gout. Ulceration with the discharge of a thick, white material (consisting of monosodium urate crystals) and superimposed infection are complications of tophaceous gout [44].

High-frequency ultrasound (US) is widely used to detect joint effusion, synovial hyperpla-

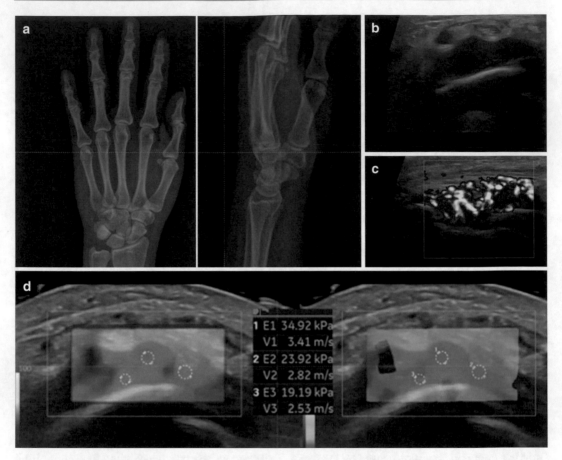

Fig. 7.7 A 54-year-old male patient with recent onset right wrist pain. The anteroposterior and lateral radiographic images (**a**) show no significant changes. Wrist ultrasonography of the wrist at the level of the dorsal radiocarpal recess shows a fair amount of articular synovial fluid (**b**). On evaluation Power Doppler mode evaluation, the synovial effusion shows diffuse vascular uptake (**c**). SWE shows increased stiffness values of the synovial fluid (**d**)

sia, and bone and articular soft tissue lesions in gouty arthritis (GA). The main typical US characteristics of GA are the double-contour sign of the articular cartilage, snowstorm appearance of the joint fluid, and hyperechoes around the periarticular tendon [48, 49]; however, it is highly challenging to distinguish GA from non-GA when the sonography results are not typical, such as in the early stage of the disease. There is where the interest in new diagnostic tools comes into place.

Tang et al. analyzed the diagnostic performance of SWE in the diagnosis of GA and non-gouty arthritis (non-GA). Based on the echo intensity of the joint lesions, the GA group was subdivided into hypo-echoic GA, slightly hyper-echoic GA, and hyper-echoic GA subgroups. When looking for parameters to differentiate GA

from non-GA they found that the elastic modulus (E_{max}), mean elastic modulus (E_{mean}), minimum elastic modulus (E_{min}), and elastic modulus standard deviation (E_{SD}) were significantly higher in the GA group than in the non-GA group and were highest in the hyper-echoic GA subgroup. E_{min}, E_{mean}, E_{max}, and E_{SD} were also higher in the hypo-echoic GA subgroup than in the non-GA group, with areas under the receiver operating curves optimal cut-off values of 29.40 kPa for E_{min}, 45.35 kPa for E_{mean}, 67.54 kPa for E_{max} and 7.85 kPa for E_{SD}. These results indicate that SWE seems to be a useful diagnostic tool to differentiate between GA and non-GA [50] (Fig. 7.7).

Fine needle biopsy (FNAB) of the effusion showed synovial fluid with diffuse accumulation of uric acid crystal deposition consistent with gout.

7.6 Thumb Osteoarthritis

The thumb basal joint is the second most common site of osteoarthritis (OA), with radiographic evidence in up to 40% of women aged >80 years and commonly affecting the non-dominant hand. Despite this high prevalence, the disease is not always clinically significant, and most patients never seek treatment. However, when symptomatic, loss of thumb function can impart up to a 50% impairment to the upper extremity. The literature suggests a range of etiologies contributing to the degeneration, including ligamentous laxity, genetics, overuse, and trauma [51].

Patients often describe activity-related pain or soreness at the base of the thumb, along with difficulty pinching and grasping. In the initial stages of osteoarthritis, an inspection of the thumb may be normal. In later stages, however, the thumb metacarpal adopts a characteristic deformity consisting of an adducted posture accompanied by a compensatory MCP hyperextension deformity. Palpation may reveal tenderness, swelling, and crepitus. Diagnosis is made with a thorough clinical examination and radiographic staging, as described by Eaton and Littler [49], although it is difficult to evaluate functional limitations and to correlate clinical and radiological findings, studies found weak relationships between the radiographic staging of first carpometacarpal (CMC) OA with functional hand performance [52–54]. As on clinical examination, CMC subluxation, metacarpal adduction, and MCP hyperextension are seen. Despite some authors note the utility of cross-sectional imaging (e.g., MRI, ultrasonography, CT) in the diagnosis of thumb basal joint arthritis, there is currently no recommended role for advanced imaging.

The role of SWE in thumb osteoarthritis has been assessed by Nwawka et al., who aimed to establish data on the SWE findings in the thenar eminence muscles in patients with first CMC OA vs healthy subjects and correlate these findings with the clinical tests of hand function. The rationale for this study was that there seems to be an interplay between the thenar eminence muscles and the ligaments which are thought to contribute to stability in the CMC joint [55] and there had

been no previous studies exploring how these changes in thenar eminence muscle quality associate with function in thumb CMC OA.

Results showed that SWE values in the abductor pollicis brevis and flexor pollicis brevis muscles showed a moderate to very strong correlation with multiple measures of hand function. Mean SWE values of the thenar eminence muscles in first CMC OA patients were lower than those in asymptomatic control subjects, meaning that patients with CMC OA have less stiff thenar eminence muscles than controls and that they correlate with decreased hand function.

7.7 Rheumatoid Arthritis

Rheumatoid arthritis (RA) is a chronic, systemic inflammatory disease that is more common in women and may occur at any age although peak incidence is between ages 50 and 60 years. The most prominent feature is symmetrical pain and swelling of the hands, wrists, feet, and knees (polyarthritis), although other joints may be affected. Patients may also present with monoarthritis or oligoarthritis.

RA should be considered in any patient with joint stiffness, pain, or swelling that persists for more than a few weeks. Joint pain in RA is typically symmetrical and polyarticular, but may be asymmetrical, oligoarticular (involving 2–4 joints), or monoarticular at the onset. Although not specific for RA, new-onset symmetrical joint swelling with morning stiffness lasting longer than an hour that improves with use throughout the day is characteristic. Synovitis is important to recognize for RA diagnosis, which is defined as an inflamed joint capsule characterized by erythema, warmth, tenderness to palpation, and swelling; it is typically detected by physical examination, but advanced imaging may be useful in patients with equivocal signs. Patients with synovitis and symptoms lasting more than 6 weeks are more likely to develop a progressive disease versus a self-limited process. Hand, wrist, and foot involvement are most common in RA, but atypical presentations may only involve large joints, such as the knee. The distal interphalangeal joints of the hand are not typically involved, and dactylitis is uncommon. The axial skeleton, including the hips, also is not typically involved, although severe and long-standing RA may involve these joints, particularly the cervical spine.

Historically, patients with longstanding, inadequately treated RA, developed joint damage and deformities, including characteristic ulnar deviation, swan neck, and boutonniere deformities of the hands and flexion contractures of the knees and elbows. Fortunately, this is not so frequent nowadays due to optimized treatment and better control of the disease [56].

There are three studies that have assessed the role of SWE in different aspects of RA.

Sammel et al., in the first pilot study of SWE in the synovium, compared synovium stiffness of patients with RA vs healthy controls and correlated SWV with disease activity. Results showed that patients with RA had lower maximum synovial SWV than controls (6.38 m/s vs. 6.99 m/s $P = 0.042$) and that there was a statistically significant negative correlation between maximum SWV and disease activity markers including gray-scale ultrasound graded synovial thickness and erythrocyte sedimentation rate. Conclusions state that further studies are warranted to confirm those observations [57].

In 2019, Alfuraih et al. investigated muscle stiffness and strength according to several exercises in RA patients compared to healthy controls. RA patients were distributed into three groups: newly diagnosed treatment-naïve RA, active RA for at least 1 year, and in remission RA

for at least 1 year. In comparison to controls, the new and active RA groups showed a significantly lower isokinetic strength by -29% ($p = 0.013$) and -28% ($p = 0.040$), fewer chair stands by -28% ($p = 0.001$) and -44% ($p < 0.001$), longer walking times by -25% ($p = 0.025$) and -30% ($p = 0.001$), respectively, and weaker grip strength by -45% for both ($p < 0.001$). SWV was not significantly different among the groups on all muscles, so although they observed significant muscle weakness in RA patients vs controls, muscle stiffness measured by SWE was normal and not associated with muscle strength in any of the groups [58].

In 2022, Chandel et al. performed another study aimed to use SWE to evaluate RA and tubercular (TB) arthritis and to differentiate them using synovial stiffness. The mean elasticity and velocity values were 54.81 ± 10.6 kPa and 4.2 m/s ± 0.42 for RA and 37 ± 10 kPa and 3.4 ± 0.47 m/s for TB group. Significant difference ($P < 0.001$) was seen in elastic modulus values between the rheumatoid and TB group with cutoff of 43.6 kPa, according to receiver operating characteristic curves, to differentiate the two groups. Similar significant ($P < 0.001$) results were seen with velocity values, with cutoff of 3.76 m/s. They conclude that SWE shows the potential to be a useful adjunct to gray-scale and color Doppler USG in differentiating various arthritis based on elastic properties of the synovium and that elastic modulus and velocity are useful SWE quantitative parameters for synovial evaluation and can differentiate RA and TB arthritis [59] (Figs. 7.8, 7.9, 7.10, and 7.11).

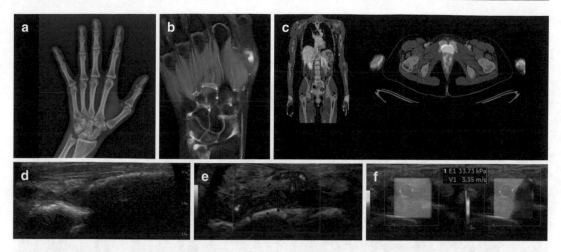

Fig. 7.8 A 30-year-old patient with RA under treatment but with persistent bilateral carpal swelling. Comparison of different imaging techniques in a patient with synovitis of right radiocarpal and intercarpal joints. (**a**) Conventional anteroposterior radiograph; (**b**) Magnetic Resonance Imaging; (**c**) Positron Emission Tomography; (**d**) B-mode Ultrasound; (**e**) Power Doppler Mode Ultrasound; (**f**) Shear Wave Elastography Mode Ultrasound

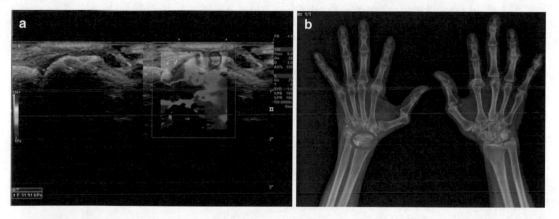

Fig. 7.9 (**a**) Increased stiffness of joint synovial tissue in the left dorsal radiocarpal joint in a 45-year-old male patient with rheumatoid arthritis showed by SWE. (**b**) Signs of nonspecific right radiocarpal arthropathy in the same patient visualized on anterior-posterior x-rays

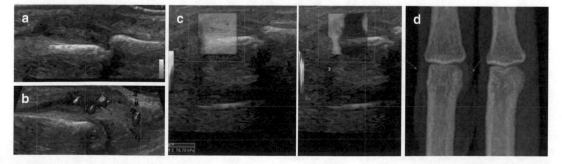

Fig. 7.10 A 37-year-old female with a history of RA. Persistent pain in the fingers was bilateral with swelling more evident in the proximal interphalangeal joints. Synovitis of the third proximal interphalangeal joint of the right hand diagnosed with: conventional ultrasound (**a**), ultrasound with Doppler module (**b**), SWE (**c**), and conventional radiograph in anteroposterior view (**d**)

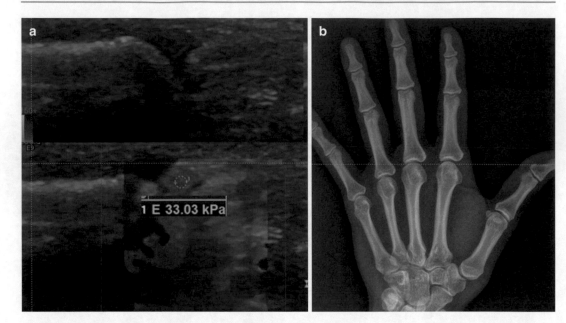

Fig. 7.11 A 51-year-old male patient with rheumatoid arthritis reporting swelling and selective pain in the second finger of the left hand. (**a**) SWE showing—Increased stiff- ness of joint synovial tissue in the left second metacarpo- phalangeal joint. (**b**) No significant radiographic changes are visible on the single-hand radiograph in AP view

7.8 Conclusion and Future Perspectives

In relation to what has been highlighted in recent years, it is evident that elastography is an almost unexplored field in the study of inflammatory joint pathology and synovitis.

We know that the sensitivity and specificity of the conventional B-Mode technique and of the vascular evaluation techniques (the most used PD) are very variable, especially as a function of the activity of the inflammatory pathology.

We believe that the evaluation with elastography, especially with the use of quantitative SWE, of the pathologies that manifest themselves with synovitis, and with subclinical or chronic synovitis, could be soon a potential tool both for early diagnosis of the disease and for monitoring the therapeutic response, and that it could suppose significant aid to the expertise of clinical colleagues.

7.9 Clinical Applications

A summary of the findings in different clinical conditions can be found in Table 7.1.

Table 7.1 Summary of SWE findings in different conditions

Clinical scenario	SWE stiffness values	Source
De Quervain's Tendinopathy	Decreased	Turkay et al. [11]
Systemic Lupus Erythematosus	Decreased in muscles	Di Matteo et al. [23]
Primary Sjögren's Syndrome	Increased	Oruk et al. [36], Arslan et al. [37], and Bădărînză et al. 2020 [46]
Gout arthritis	Increased	Tang et al. [50]
Thumb Osteoarthritis	Decreased in thenar eminence muscles in first CMC	Nwawka et al. [55]
Reumathoid Arthritis	Decreased in a comparative study with healthy subjects (Sammel) - increased in a comparative study between RA and Tuberculous arthritis (Chandel)	Sammel et al. [57] and Chandel et al. [59]

References

1. Patil P, Dasgupta B. Role of diagnostic ultrasound in the assessment of musculoskeletal diseases. Ther Adv Musculoskelet Dis. 2012;4(5):341–55.
2. Gabba A, Piga M, Vacca A, Porru G, Garau P, Cauli A, et al. Joint and tendon involvement in systemic lupus erythematosus: an ultrasound study of hands and wrists in 108 patients. Rheumatol (United Kingdom). 2012;51(12):2278–85.
3. Burke CJ, Alizai H, Beltran LS, Regatte RR. MRI of synovitis and joint fluid. J Magn Reson Imaging. 2019;49(6):1512–27.
4. D'Agostino MA, Terslev L, Aegerter P, Backhaus M, Balint P, Bruyn GA, et al. Scoring ultrasound synovitis in rheumatoid arthritis: a EULAR-OMERACT ultrasound taskforce - Part 1: definition and development of a standardised, consensus-based scoring system. RMD Open. 2017;3(1):e00428.
5. Costantino F, Carmona L, Boers M, Backhaus M, Balint PV, Bruyn GA, et al. EULAR recommendations for the reporting of ultrasound studies in rheumatic and musculoskeletal diseases (RMDs). Ann Rheum Dis. 2021;80(7):840–7.
6. Snoj Ž, Wu CH, Taljanovic MS, Dumić-Čule I, Drakonaki EE, Klauser AS. Ultrasound elastography in musculoskeletal radiology: past, present, and future. Semin Musculoskelet Radiol. 2020;24(2):156–66.
7. Schumacher HR Jr, Dorwart BB, Korzeniowski OM. Occurrence of De Quervain's tendinitis during pregnancy. Arch Intern Med. 1985;145:2083.
8. Anderson BC. Office orthopedics for primary care: diagnosis and treatment. 2nd ed. Philadelphia: WB Saunders; 1999.
9. Clarke MT, Lyall HA, Grant JW, Matthewson MH. The histopathology of de Quervain's disease. J Hand Surg Br. 1998;23:732.
10. Sato J, Ishii Y, Noguchi H. Clinical and ultrasound features in patients with intersection syndrome or de Quervain's disease. J Hand Surg Eur. 2016;41:220.
11. Turkay R, Inci E, Aydeniz B, Vural M. Shear wave elastography findings of de Quervain tenosynovitis. Eur J Radiol. 2017;95:192–6. https://doi.org/10.1016/j.ejrad.2017.08.011. Epub 2017 Aug 18.
12. D'Cruz DP, Kamastha MA, Huges GRV. Systemic lupus erythematosus. Lancet. 2007;369:587–96.
13. Hopkinson ND, Doherty M, Powell RJ. Clinical features and race-specific incidence/prevalence rates of systemic lupus erythematosus in a geographically complete cohort of patients. Ann Rheum Dis. 1994;53:675–80.
14. Gudmundsson S, Steinsson K. Systemic lupus erythematosus in Iceland 1975 through 1984. A nationwide epidemiological study in an unselected population. J Rheumatol. 1990;17:1162–7.
15. Johnson AE, Gordon C, Palmer RG, Bacon PA. The prevalence and incidence of systemic lupus erythematosus in Birmingham, England. Relationship to ethnicity and country of birth. Arthritis Rheum. 1995;38:551–8.
16. Seoane-Mato D, Sánchez-Piedra C, Silva-Fernández L, Sivera F, Blanco FJ, Pérez Ruiz F, Juan-Mas A, Pego-Reigosa JM, Narváez J, Quilis Martí N, Cortés Verdú R, Antón-Pagés F, Quevedo Vila V, Garrido Courel L, Del Amo NDV, Paniagua Zudaire I, Añez Sturchio G, Medina Varo F, Ruiz Tudela MDM, Romero Pérez A, Ballina J, Brandy García A, Fábregas Canales D, Font Gayá T, Bordoy Ferrer C, González Álvarez B, Casas Hernández L, Álvarez Reyes F, Delgado Sánchez M, Martínez Dubois C, Sánchez-Fernández SÁ, Rojas Vargas LM, García Morales PV, Olivé A, Rubio Muñoz P, Larrosa M, Navarro Ricos N, Graell Martín E, Chamizo E, Chaves Chaparro L, Rojas Herrera S, Pons Dolset J, Polo Ostariz MÁ, Ruiz-Alejos Garrido S, Macía Villa C, Cruz Valenciano A, González Gómez ML, Morcillo Valle M, Palma Sánchez D, Moreno Martínez MJ, Mayor González M, Atxotegi Sáenz de Buruaga J, Urionagüena Onaindia I, Blanco Cáceres BA, Díaz-González F, Bustabad S. Prevalence of rheumatic diseases in adult population in Spain (EPISER 2016 study): aims and methodology. Reumatol Clin (Engl Ed). 2019;15(2):90–6. https://doi.org/10.1016/j.reuma.2017.06.009.
17. Crispín JC, Liossis SN, Kis-Toth K, Lieberman LA, Kyttaris VC, Juang YT, Tsokos GC. Pathogenesis of human systemic lupus erythematosus: recent advances. Trends Mol Med. 2010;16:47–57.
18. Cervera R, Abarca-Costalago M, Abramovicz D, Allegri F, Annunziata P, Aydintug AO, Bacarelli MR, Bellisai F, Bernardino I, Biernat-Kaluza E, Blockmans D, Boki K, Bracci L, Campanella V, Camps MT, Carcassi C, Cattaneo R, Cauli A, Chwalinska-Sadowska H, Contu L, Cosyns JP, Danieli MG, D'Cruz D, Depresseux G, Direskeneli H, Domènech I, Espinosa G, Fernández-Nebro A, Ferrara GB, Font J, Frutos MA, Galeazzi M, García-Carrasco M, García-Iglesias MF, García-Tobaruela A, George J, Gil A, González-Santos P, Grana M, Gül A, Haga HJ, de Haro-Liger M, Houssiau F, Hughes GR, Ingelmo M, Jedryka-Góral A, Khamashta MA, Lavilla P, Levi Y, López-Dupla M, López-Soto A, Maldykowa H, Marcolongo R, Mathieu A, Morozzi G, Nicolopoulou N, Papasteriades C, Passiu G, Perelló I, Petera P, Petrovic R, Piette JC, Pintado V, de Pita O, Popovic R, Pucci G, Puddu P, de Ramón E, Ramos-Casals M, Rodríguez-Andreu J, Ruiz-Irastroza G, Sánchez-Lora J, Sanna G, Scorza R, Sebastini GD, Sherer Y, Shoenfeld Y, Simpatico A, Sinico RA, Smolen J, Tincani A, Tokgöz G, Urbano-Márquez A, Vasconcelos C, Vázquez JJ, Veronesi M, Vianni J, Vivancos J, European Working Party on Systemic Lupus Erythematosus. Lessons from the "Euro-Lupus Cohort". Ann Med Interne (Paris). 2002;153(8):530–6.
19. Carrión-Barberà I, Salman-Monte TC, Vílchez-Oya F, Monfort J. Neuropsychiatric involvement in systemic lupus erythematosus: a review. Autoimmun Rev. 2021;20(4):102780. https://doi.org/10.1016/j.autrev.2021.102780. Epub 2021 Feb 18.

20. Hochberg MC. Updating the American College of Rheumatology revised criteria for the classification of systemic lupus erythematosus. Arthritis Rheum. 1997;40:1725.

21. Petri M, Orbai AM, Alarcón GS, Gordon C, Merrill JT, Fortin PR, Bruce IN, Isenberg D, Wallace DJ, Nived O, Sturfelt G, Ramsey-Goldman R, Bae SC, Hanly JG, Sánchez-Guerrero J, Clarke A, Aranow C, Manzi S, Urowitz M, Gladman D, Kalunian K, Costner M, Werth VP, Zoma A, Bernatsky S, Ruiz-Irastorza G, Khamashta MA, Jacobsen S, Buyon JP, Maddison P, Dooley MA, van Vollenhoven RF, Ginzler E, Stoll T, Peschken C, Jorizzo JL, Callen JP, Lim SS, Fessler BJ, Inanc M, Kamen DL, Rahman A, Steinsson K, Franks AG Jr, Sigler L, Hameed S, Fang H, Pham N, Brey R, Weisman MH, McGwin G Jr, Magder LS. Derivation and validation of the systemic lupus international collaborating clinics classification criteria for systemic lupus erythematosus. Arthritis Rheum. 2012;64:2677–86.

22. Aringer M, Costenbader K, Daikh D, Brinks R, Mosca M, Ramsey-Goldman R, Smolen JS, Wofsy D, Boumpas DT, Kamen DL, Jayne D, Cervera R, Costedoat-Chalumeau N, Diamond B, Gladman DD, Hahn B, Hiepe F, Jacobsen S, Khanna D, Lerstrøm K, Massarotti E, McCune J, Ruiz-Irastorza G, Sanchez-Guerrero J, Schneider M, Urowitz M, Bertsias G, Hoyer BF, Leuchten N, Tani C, Tedeschi SK, Touma Z, Schmajuk G, Anic B, Assan F, Chan TM, Clarke AE, Crow MK, Czirják L, Doria A, Graninger W, Halda-Kiss B, Hasni S, Izmirly PM, Jung M, Kumánovics G, Mariette X, Padjen I, Pego-Reigosa JM, Romero-Diaz J, Rúa-Figueroa Fernández Í, Seror R, Stummvoll GH, Tanaka Y, Tektonidou MG, Vasconcelos C, Vital EM, Wallace DJ, Yavuz S, Meroni PL, Fritzler MJ, Naden R, Dörner T, Johnson SR. 2019 European League Against Rheumatism/American College of Rheumatology classification criteria for systemic lupus erythematosus. Ann Rheum Dis. 2019;78(9):1151–9. https://doi.org/10.1136/annrheumdis-2018-214819. Epub 2019 Aug 5.

23. Di Matteo A, Smerilli G, Cipolletta E, Wakefield RJ, De Angelis R, Risa AM, Salaffi F, Farah S, Villota-Eraso C, Maccarone V, Filippucci E, Grassi W. Muscle involvement in systemic lupus erythematosus: multimodal ultrasound assessment and relationship with physical performance. Rheumatology (Oxford). 2022:keac196. https://doi.org/10.1093/rheumatology/keac196. Epub ahead of print.

24. Torrente-Segarra V, Salman-Monte TC, Corominas H. Musculoskeletal involvement and ultrasonography update in systemic lupus erythematosus: new insights and review. Eur J Rheumatol. 2018;5:127–30.

25. Zayat AS, Md Yusof MY, Wakefield RJ, Conaghan PG, Emery P, Vital EM. The role of ultrasound in assessing musculoskeletal symptoms of systemic lupus erythematosus: a systematic literature review. Rheumatology (Oxford). 2016;55:485–94. 14.

26. Wong PC, Lee G, Sedie AD, Hanova P, Inanc N, Jousse-Joulin S, et al. Musculoskeletal ultrasound in systemic lupus erythematosus: systematic literature review by the lupus task force of the OMERACT Ultrasound Working Group. J Rheumatol. 2019;46:1379–87.

27. Bowman SJ. Primary Sjögren's syndrome. Lupus. 2018;27:32–5.

28. Qin B, Wang J, Yang Z, Yang M, Ma N, Huang F, et al. Epidemiology of primary Sjögren síndrome: a systematic review and meta-analysis. Ann Rheum Dis. 2015;74:1983–9.

29. Ramos-Casals M, Solans R, Rosas J, Camps MT, Gil A, del Pino-Montes J, et al. Primary Sjögren síndrome in Spain. Clinical and immunologic expression in 1010 patients. Medicine. 2008;87:210–9.

30. Fernández Castro M, Andreu JL, Sanchez-Piedra C, Martínez Taboada V, Olivé A, Rosas J, et al. SJOGREN-SER: registro nacional de pacientes con síndrome de Sjögren primario de la Sociedad Española de Reumatología, objetivos y metodología. Reumatol Clin. 2016;12:184–9.

31. Botsios C, Furlan A, Ostuni P, Sfriso P, Andretta M, Ometto F, et al. Elderly onset of primary Sjögren's syndrome: clinical manifestations, serological features and oral/ocular diagnostic tests. Comparison with adult and young onset of the disease in a cohort of 336 Italian patients. Jt Bone Spine. 2011;78:171–4.

32. Seror R, Theander E, Brun JG, et al. Validation of EULAR primary Sjögren's syndrome disease activity (ESSDAI) and patient indexes (ESSPRI). Ann Rheum Dis. 2015;74:859–66.

33. Seror R, Ravaud P, Mariette X, et al. EULAR Sjögren's syndrome patient reported index (ESSPRI): development of a consensus patient index for primary Sjogren's syndrome. Ann Rheum Dis. 2011;70:968–72.

34. Ramos-Casals M, Brito-Zerón P, Bombardieri S, Bootsma H, De Vita S, Dörner T, Fisher BA, Gottenberg JE, Hernandez-Molina G, Kocher A, Kostov B, Kruize AA, Mandl T, Ng WF, Retamozo S, Seror R, Shoenfeld Y, Sisó-Almirall A, Tzioufas AG, Vitali C, Bowman S, Mariette X, EULAR-Sjögren Syndrome Task Force Group. EULAR recommendations for the management of Sjögren's syndrome with topical and systemic therapies. Ann Rheum Dis. 2020;79(1):3–18. https://doi.org/10.1136/annrheumdis-2019-216,114. Epub 2019 Oct 31.

35. Shiboski CH, Shiboski SC, Seror R, Criswell LA, Labetoulle M, Lietman TM, Rasmussen A, Scofield H, Vitali C, Bowman SJ, Mariette X, International Sjögren's Syndrome Criteria Working Group. 2016 American College of Rheumatology/European league against rheumatism classification criteria for primary Sjögren's syndrome: a consensus and data-driven methodology involving three international patient cohorts. Arthritis Rheumatol. 2017;69(1):35–45. https://doi.org/10.1002/art.39859. Epub 2016 Oct 26.

36. Oruk YE, Çildağ MB, Karaman CZ, Çildağ S. Effectiveness of ultrasonography and shear wave sonoelastography in Sjögren syndrome with

salivary gland involvement. Ultrasonography. 2021;40(4):584–93. https://doi.org/10.14366/usg.21014. Epub 2021 Mar 23.

37. Arslan S, Durmaz MS, Erdogan H, Esmen SE, Turgut B, Iyisoy MS. Two-dimensional shear wave elastography in the assessment of salivary gland involvement in primary Sjögren's syndrome. J Ultrasound Med. 2020;39(5):949–56. https://doi.org/10.1002/jum.15179. Epub 2019 Nov 25.

38. Hocevar A, Ambrozic A, Rozman B, Kveder T, Tomsic M. Ultrasonographic changes of major salivary glands in primary Sjogren's syndrome. Diagnostic value of a novel scoring system. Rheumatology (Oxford). 2005;44(6):768–72. https://doi.org/10.1093/rheumatology/keh588. Epub 2005 Mar 1.

39. Milic VD, Petrovic RR, Boricic IV, Radunovic GL, Pejnovic NN, Soldatovic I, Damjanov NS. Major salivary gland sonography in Sjögren's syndrome: diagnostic value of a novel ultrasonography score (0–12) for parenchymal inhomogeneity. Scand J Rheumatol. 2010;39(2):160–6. https://doi.org/10.3109/03009740903270623.

40. Jousse-Joulin S, Nowak E, Cornec D, Brown J, Carr A, Carotti M, Fisher B, Fradin J, Hocevar A, Jonsson MV, Luciano N, Milic V, Rout J, Theander E, Stel A, Bootsma H, Vissink A, Baldini C, Baer A, Ng WF, Bowman S, Alavi Z, Saraux A, Devauchelle-Pensec V. Salivary gland ultrasound abnormalities in primary Sjögren's syndrome: consensual US-SG core items definition and reliability. RMD Open. 2017;3(1):e000364. https://doi.org/10.1136/rmdopen-2016-000364.

41. De Vita S, Lorenzon G, Rossi G, Sabella M, Fossaluzza V. Salivary gland echography in primary and secondary Sjogren's syndrome. Clin Exp Rheumatol. 1992;10:351–6. pmid:1395220.

42. Makula E, Pokorny G, Rajtár M, Kiss I, Kovács A, Kovács L. Parotid gland ultrasonography as a diagnostic tool in primary Sjögren's syndrome. Br J Rheumatol. 1996;35(10):972–7. https://doi.org/10.1093/rheumatology/35.10.972.

43. Wernicke D, Hess H, Gromnica-Ihle E, Krause A, Schmidt WA. Ultrasonography of salivary glands—a highly specific imaging procedure for diagnosis of Sjögren's syndrome. J Rheumatol. 2008;35(2):285–93. Epub 2008 Jan 15.

44. Salaffi F, Carotti M, Iagnocco A, Luccioli F, Ramonda R, Sabatini E, De Nicola M, Maggi M, Priori R, Valesini G, Gerli R, Punzi L, Giuseppetti GM, Salvolini U, Grassi W. Ultrasonography of salivary glands in primary Sjögren's syndrome: a comparison with contrast sialography and scintigraphy. Rheumatology (Oxford). 2008;47(8):1244–9. https://doi.org/10.1093/rheumatology/ken222. Epub 2008 Jun 19.

45. Theander E, Mandl T. Primary Sjögren's syndrome: diagnostic and prognostic value of salivary gland ultrasonography using a simplified scoring system. Arthritis Care Res (Hoboken). 2014;66(7):1102–7. https://doi.org/10.1002/acr.22264.

46. Bădărînză M, Serban O, Maghear L, Bocsa C, Micu M, Damian L, Felea I, Fodor D. Shear wave elastography as a new method to identify parotid lymphoma in primary Sjögren syndrome patients: an observational study. Rheumatol Int. 2020;40(8):1275–81. https://doi.org/10.1007/s00296-020-04548-x. Epub 2020 Mar 21.

47. Dalbeth N, Gosling AL, Gaffo A, Abhishek A. Gout. Lancet. 2021;10(287):1843–55.

48. Chowalloor PV, Keen HI. A systematic review of ultrasonography in gout and asymptomatic hyperuricaemia. Ann Rheum Dis. 2013;72:638–45.

49. Leng QY, Tang YJ, Zhang LY, Xiang X, Qiu L, Su BH. Diagnostic value of ultrasound imaging in chronic gouty arthritis. J Sichuan Univ (Medical Sci Ed). 2014;45:424–7.

50. Tang Y, Yan F, Yang Y, Xiang X, Wang L, Zhang L, Qiu L. Value of shear wave elastography in the diagnosis of gouty and non-gouty arthritis. Ultrasound Med Biol. 2017;43:884–92.

51. Weiss APC, Goodman AD. Thumb basal joint arthritis. J Am Acad Orthop Surg. 2018;26:562–71.

52. Dahaghin S, Bierma-Zeinstra SMA, Ginai AZ, Pols HAP, Hazes JMW, Koes BW. Prevalence and pattern of radiographic hand osteoarthritis and association with pain and disability (the Rotterdam study). Ann Rheum Dis. 2005;64:682–7.

53. Haugen IK, Slatkowsky-Christensen B, Bøyesen P, van der Heijde D, Kvien TK. Cross-sectional and longitudinal associations between radiographic features and measures of pain and physical function in hand osteoarthritis. Osteoarthr Cartil. 2013;21:1191–8.

54. Hoffler CE, Matzon JL, Lutsky KF, Kim N, Beredjiklian PK. Radiographic stage does not correlate with symptom severity in thumb basilar joint osteoarthritis. J Am Acad Orthop Surg. 2015;23:778–82.

55. Nwawka OK, Weinstock-Zlotnick G, Lin B, Ko LM. Association of clinical assessments of hand function and quantitative ultrasound metrics in first carpometacarpal osteoarthritis. HSS J. 2020;16(Suppl 2):420–4. https://doi.org/10.1007/s11420-020-09795-z. Epub 2020 Sep 29.

56. Sparks JA. In the Clinic® rheumatoid arthritis. Ann Intern Med. 2019;170:ITC1.

57. Sammel AM, Spies MC, DeCarle R, Rayment M, Joshua F. Shear-wave elastographic ultrasound of metacarpophalangeal synovium in rheumatoid arthritis - a pilot study. Australas J Ultrasound Med. 2017;20:58–65.

58. Alfuraih AM, Tan AL, O'Connor P, Emery P, Wakefield RJ. Muscle stiffness in rheumatoid arthritis is not altered or associated with muscle weakness: a shear wave elastography study. Mod Rheumatol. 2020;30:617–25.

59. Chandel K, Prakash M, Sinha A, Sharma A, Chouhan DK, Sandhu MS. Role of shear wave elastography of synovium to differentiate rheumatoid and tubercular arthritis. J Med Ultrasound. 2022;30:30.

Printed in the United States
by Baker & Taylor Publisher Services